THE ART OF LOOKING YOUNGER

The ageing skin has always been a source of great concern to human beings, and there is a long recorded history of attempts to improve or correct it. A medical papyrus, written by an unknown Egyptian over three thousand years ago, describes some of these early efforts. If you had been born in ancient Egypt, your sole weapon against ageing would have been a facial masque of dubious value. Now you have help that was not available in those days, even to Pharaoh himself.

This book can help you plan an effective up-to-date programme for the total care of your appearance, one that exactly suits your personal needs. The time to begin is now.

The Art of Looking Younger

Dr Bedford Shelmire

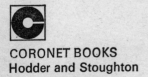

CORONET BOOKS
Hodder and Stoughton

First published in Great Britain 1974 by
David & Charles (Holdings) Limited

Coronet Edition 1976

Printed and bound in Great Britain for
Coronet Books, Hodder and Stoughton London,
By Richard Clay (The Chaucer Press), Ltd.,
Bungay, Suffolk

ISBN 0 340 21008 7

CONTENTS

ONE

PROLOGUE

'Every man desires to live long, but no man would be old.'
Swift, *Thoughts on Various Subjects*

The aging skin has always been a source of great concern to human beings, and there is a long recorded history of attempts to improve or correct it. A medical papyrus, written by an unknown Egyptian over three thousand years ago, describes some of these early efforts. It includes a formula for 'transforming an old man into a youth'; and the preamble enthusiastically states it will 'beautify the skin, remove wrinkles from the head, remove blemishes, disfigurements, and all signs of age.' For the still unconvinced, the pitch ends with a line that would put a modern copywriter to shame, stating simply that the formula will 'remove all weaknesses which are in the flesh.' The Egyptian must have also been a skilled chemist, because the recipe would make any modern pharmacist reach for the nearest bottle of tranquillizers. The active ingredient was something called hemayet-fruit, apparently not a common staple even in that day, for it has never been positively identified. After a lengthy and complicated mixing procedure, done only in certain specified containers, the preparation was applied directly to the skin, where it was allowed to dry. As the moisture evaporated into the warm, dry air of the Nile Valley, there was at first a cooling sensation, which must have been very soothing to sunbaked, sand-blasted skin. As the drying proceeded a bit further, the skin began to feel drawn and constricted. Finally, the preparation was rinsed off, leaving behind a clean, refreshed-feeling skin. Sound familiar? It should, at least to most women, because the Egyptian had invented the first facial masque. This certainly doesn't put him right up there with Pasteur and Salk, but it was an innovation at the time. Later on, the Greeks and Romans used mudpacks for the same purposes and, surprisingly enough, masques very similar to the original are sold today at every cosmetic counter.

As a matter of fact, we have only recently acquired the ability to really do something about the more serious changes in appearance that accompany aging. Although the truth of this statement is beyond dispute, it does raise a question. Haven't there been many people throughout the course of history who were famous for their timeless and unchanging faces? Yes, there certainly have been such people, and their remarkable physical attributes are well documented in a number of cases. Long before the scientific era, there were great beauties whose durable good looks inspired volumes of poetry and prose. In more recent times, there were the entertainers and 'society' figures of the last century. Many of these notables are remembered as much for their indestructible features as they are for their accomplishments. How did they do it? Certainly not with mudpacks and fruit masques and, as we shall see, they didn't discover any secret formulas, as some cosmetic companies would have you believe. Prior to the scientific era, there were only two ways to a younger appearance: constant pampering of the skin or sheer accident.

This requires a word of explanation. The very wealthy, with the time and money to take care of themselves, have always looked better than their overworked, poverty-ridden contemporaries. There are, however, definite limits to what any amount of unenlightened pampering can accomplish, and I suspect that many of these celebrated personages also had an assist from heredity. About one person in a thousand inherits genes that seem to insure a practically ageproof skin, regardless of the care given. This kind of happy genetic accident is a much more important factor in determining how well any particular face resists the ravages of time.

In the past, the average person stood very little chance of being able to look younger. Without wealth or the right genes, there was very little hope. The advent of modern skin care has changed all this. Now, it is no longer necessary to constantly pamper yourself or be born with a good skin. The idle rich no longer have any advantage, because modern skin care is well within the reach of everyone. It takes only a few minutes a day, and the products needed are inexpensive and easily obtainable. The genes you inherit are no longer a limiting factor, because we can now compensate for even delicate, age-prone skin. Your bank account or family tree no longer makes much difference. Thanks to modern research, we now know what causes many of the unattractive problems that appear with age. With this kind of knowledge, we have been able to develop methods that are effective in combating or solving these problems.

The practical application of these methods can produce spectacular results. A person can easily look ten or twenty years younger than his or her actual age, and this can be achieved with a minimum of effort. My own interest in this subject was first stimulated by an eminent dermatologist who was one of my first teachers. He was not only an early advocate of these new methods, but he also practised them himself. The results were truly impressive. At almost eighty years of age, he appeared to be in his early fifties.

Since starting my own practice, I have constantly tried to teach these methods to patients, friends, and anyone else who would listen. As the years have gone by, those who have taken this advice are increasingly glad they did. In terms of personal satisfaction, there is no doubt that good skin care is one of today's best bargains. I can think of nothing else that gives such high returns on such a small investment of time and effort.

Before discussing these methods in detail, it is essential that the reader have some understanding of their development. The modern approach to the skin's aging problems is based on using not one, but two separate and distinct types of care. These two types of care differ from each other in many important respects, and are called corrective skin care and preventive skin care. Together, they represent the foundation of the modern approach, and we shall refer to them again and again throughout the ensuing pages.

Corrective skin care involves the repair of aging skin, and corrective action is taken only after the aging changes appear. This type of care has been practised in one form or another since time immemorial. When some 'over-thirty' Neanderthal saw his reflection in a pond or stream and noticed a fresh crop of wrinkles, it is probably safe to assume that his first impulse was to find a way to remove them. What he did, of course, we shall never know. Later on, we have the primitive attempts at corrective care made by the Egyptian and his successors. Corrective care has undergone so many evolutions and improvements that the modern version would be almost unrecognizable to these early practitioners. However, the basic concept has remained unchanged since the beginning.

Preventive care is the newer of these two types of care and potentially the more important. As the name implies, its purpose is to anticipate and prevent aging changes. Recent studies have shown that many skin problems can be completely avoided by taking a few simple precautions, something unheard of a few years ago. The most significant difference between corrective and preventive care is the timing of each. In corrective care, the time element is relatively unimportant; the results are the same regardless of when it is started—whether in adolescence, last year, or yesterday. Preventive care is altogether different.

Here, the time element is very important, and the earlier preventive care is begun, the better for long-term results. Corrective care is accepted more readily because it fulfils an immediate need; it also produces more immediate results. The need for preventive care is just as great, but, since it isn't obvious in the earlier years, the fact that the need exists at all must be accepted on faith. However, both types of care must be pursued with equal vigour if the skin is ever to achieve its full potential.

We will begin our search for a younger appearance by discussing some of the scientific facts from which the principles of corrective and preventive care are derived. We will then be ready to discuss in detail the practical aspects of modern skin care. First and foremost is what you do for yourself, or personal skin care. Here we will not only discuss methods but the specific products you should use. We will try to cut through the mumbo jumbo, abracadabra, and sometimes pure nonsense that surrounds the selling of skin-care products. We will tell you what kinds of products are available for each particular skin and its problems, what these products contain, and why some work much better than others. We will also prove to you that good skin care needn't be expensive and try to help you avoid paying exorbitant prices for inferior or useless merchandise. There are inexpensive substitutes for many skin-care products, and these 'home remedies' are in some cases more effective than the high-priced products sold in cosmetic departments. We'll tell you about these, too.

In addition to personal skin care, we will see what

other people, such as dermatologists, cosmetologists, medical specialists and plastic surgeons can do to help you. We will have something to say about the roles of such things as foods and vitamins, and the effect of weight changes. We will also explore the relationship between an individual's appearance and his or her particular life style. To complete the picture, there will be a chapter on the hair, hands, and nails.

This book can help you plan an effective up-to-date programme for the total care of your appearance, one that exactly suits your personal needs. The time to begin is now, since the effects of a long lifetime of neglect and abuse can never be completely reversed. But think how lucky you are! If you had been born in ancient Egypt, your sole weapon against aging would have been a facial masque of dubious value. Now you have help that was not available in those days, even to Pharaoh himself.

TWO

THE SKIN AND ITS PROBLEMS

'The time will come when it will vex you to look at a mirror, and grief will prove a second cause of wrinkles.'

Ovid, *De Medicamine*

Many books have been written on skin care, but most of them fall into two distinct groups. Either they are treatises written by professionals dealing with the care of normal skin, or they are written to propound the theories and promote the fads of zealous amateurs. The first type of book is interesting and informative within limits, but we are primarily concerned here with the problems caused by aging; in this sense, the skin is never really 'normal' from the day of birth. The second type of book always approaches the problem of aging from the inside out, assuming that if you treat the rest of your body well, the attached skin will automatically reap the benefits. The most frequently encountered programmes involve special diets, and I still occasionally stumble across the bleached literary bones of some long-forgotten food faddist in a corner of the public library. (The beauty of this dietetic approach is that it is foolproof—for its propounder. The diets are invariably impossible to stick to, providing a perfect alibi for their failure to produce results.)

This book will confine itself exclusively to the problems encountered by the skin as it ages, the structural changes that cause them, and how they can affect your appearance. Before discussing specific solutions, however, we should first have a thorough understanding of how these problems originate. This means becoming familiar with both the structure and function of the skin, and learning how they are affected by the passage of time.

The skin is an organ of the body, like the liver or heart, but it differs from internal organs in several important respects. The most obvious difference is location; it's right out there where everyone can see its condition. You may be running on one kidney or only a small piece of liver, but no one will ever know the difference unless you actually keel over. Every square inch of skin counts as far as the appearance is concerned, and, like minor damage to a fine painting, a few flaws can ruin the overall effect.

The trouble is, unfortunately, that skin shows its age more than any other organ. In view of its importance to our sense of well-being, it seems a shame that something tucked away like the appendix couldn't bear this burden. An eighty-year-old bone looks pretty much like a twenty-year-old bone, but a comparison of young and old facial skin shows dramatic differences.

One reason the skin ages faster than any other organ is that its external location makes it highly vulnerable to attack. Although we often tend to think of our skin as a piece of personal decor, it is a functional organ, and it is there to encase and protect the rest of the body. Like any protective covering, it represents a first line of defence and has to take a lot of hard knocks. If this wear and tear is allowed to proceed unchecked, damage will always result. This explains why the skin is the only bodily organ requiring regular care throughout life to maintain its appearance. If you neglect any part of this care, the skin will eventually retaliate by developing wrinkles.

Since there is such a striking change in the skin's appearance from birth to old age, you would logically expect to find some equally impressive changes in its structure and function. These do indeed occur, and a comparison between young and old skin can furnish certain important keys to our understanding of what we must do to keep the skin looking as young as possible.

The skin can be divided into two layers: the outer layer, which you see, and an inner, supporting layer, which you don't see. The outer layer's primary function is to provide physical protection for the inner layer. In addition, the outer layer also acts as a highly efficient barrier. In this capacity, it not only seals in all the body's fluids, but it keeps a number of potentially harmful things out of the system. Substances that can penetrate the outer layer are easily absorbed into the general circulation, and only a very few chemicals and drugs have this special ability. The inner layer, in return for all these favours, supports the outer layer, nourishes it, and supplies it with that most important commodity—moisture.

From our standpoint, the anatomical structure of

the two layers is even more interesting than their function. As time goes by, specific structural changes occur in each layer, and the sum of these changes is what produces the appearance of age. The two layers are very dissimilar in structure, and a brief analogy may be helpful in understanding the implications of these age changes. The outer layer can be compared to the exterior of a house, and the inner layer to its foundation. Minor damage to the exterior, such as weathering of the paint or trim, decreases the attractiveness of the house, but restoration is usually not too difficult. The supporting foundation, although not visible from the outside, is still vital to the overall appearance of the house. Here, damage can have more serious effects. Cracks may appear in the outside walls, and the whole structure may sag badly, or even collapse. A bad foundation is much more difficult to repair than a worn exterior, and, if the damage is too extensive, a complete rebuilding will be necessary. The situation is almost exactly the same with the skin's outer and inner layers. If outer layer damage has not gone too far, partial or complete restoration is usually feasible. It is almost impossible to restore the inner layer, and here we must plan ahead and try to prevent damage.

The outer layer consists of several rows of living cells covered by multiple sheets of densely compacted dead cells. This layer is constantly growing, just like the related structures of hair and nail. The living cells are born at the base of the outer layer. They quickly die, and the dead cells are then pushed toward the outer surface of the skin by the arrival of new, living cells. If you remove a portion of the outer layer, it will grow back as good as new, much as a hair will grow back if cut off flush with the scalp. Think of all the millions of cuts, nicks, and superficial scratches this layer receives during a lifetime! If the injury is limited to the outer layer, complete replacement always occurs, and the damaged area heals without a trace of scar.

The dead cells of the outer layer are less strongly stuck together than those of hair and nails, and are continually shedding at the surface. This process serves several useful functions. For one thing, it gets rid of the older and drier cells. It also acts as a self-cleansing mechanism, causing bacteria, dirt, air pollutants, and other potentially harmful substances on the skin surface to be cast off.

The metabolic requirements of the living and dead cells of the outer layer are entirely different. The living reproductive cells are nourished by the general circulation, via the inner layer, and their requirements are the same as those of any other living tissue. The dead cells, which make up the greater part of the outer layer, have only one requirement, and that is water. This is the only thing in the world that will plump up these cells and soften them. A piece of dry skin can be soaked for a century in any oil or grease known to man, including the secretions of the skin's oil or sebaceous glands, and it will not soften one iota. If a few drops of water are added, however, it immediately becomes soft and pliable. Water and water alone is the only thing that can actually soften the skin—it is the ultimate moisturizer.

Oils, greases, and similar substances, by virtue of common and generally accepted usage, are called 'moisturizers,' but they don't physically moisturize the skin, they only *promote* moisturization by sealing in the available water. This distinction is highly important. It was first demonstrated experimentally by taking thin slices of dead tissue pared from the tops of corns (or bunions) on the feet and then soaking them in a variety of substances. None of the substances previously thought to be moisturizers would soften these hard strips of tissue—only water was capable of doing this. If you have a sharp razor blade and corns on your feet (or can borrow a couple from someone who does), you can repeat this very basic experiment in the privacy of your own home. Understanding and accepting the mechanics and terminology of moisturization is not always easy, and the subject is so important that it will be covered again in more detail in the chapter on moisturization.

The amount of moisture or water the outside layer holds is a major factor in determining the skin's texture, and is also responsible for some aspects of its contour. The amount of water held by these dead cells determines whether the skin surface is soft, smooth, and even; or dry, rough, and covered with fine, crepey lines. Although the outer layer receives a steady supply of water from the inner layer, the amount that can be delivered in any given period is strictly limited. This means that the outer layer is often short of water. If the loss to the atmosphere exceeds the supply, which can happen under certain atmospheric conditions, the outer layer may suddenly find itself in danger of going completely dry. This situation is analogous to a man trying to cross a desert with only one canteen. He might make it under highly favourable conditions, but any adverse change in the environment will quickly exhaust his water supply. Obviously, both the skin and the traveller should have an alternate source of moisture in addition to their fixed rations. Otherwise, they might soon find themselves in serious trouble.

The outer layer is also the source of the skin's pigment. This gives the skin its colour, and, as we all know, the amount of pigment increases when the skin is exposed to sunlight. This tanning is one of the skin's protective responses and serves to shield the delicate inner layer. Much of this increase is temporary, but part of it may be permanent, as we shall see.

The hair roots, oil glands, and sweat glands also belong to the outer layer. They actually lie below this layer, but they communicate with it by means of tubular ducts. Of these three accessory structures, the oil glands have the most direct influence on the skin's well-being. The surface ends of the oil gland ducts are commonly called pores.

The inner layer is quite different from the outer, and it plays a much greater part in determining the skin's contour. This layer cannot regenerate or replace itself, and will grow only until physical maturity is reached. Damage to the inner layer results in degeneration and the formation of scar tissue, so any injury to it, however slight, will cause a permanent structural change. In addition to contour, this layer is also responsible for tone and resiliency; its condition determines whether the skin is taut and unlined or wrinkled, loose, and sagging. The tissue of this layer is all living. It consists of bundles of tough supporting tissue interlaced with elastic fibres. The composition somewhat resembles reinforced concrete, another widely used structural material. The inner layer further contains all of the skin's blood vessels. These not only transport water and nutrients to the entire skin, but play an important secondary role in setting the colour tone of the complexion.

This has been a description of young skin, or skin as it should be in everyone, regardless of age. If we examine older skin that has been neglected or abused, we find some very startling differences.

The most important structural changes found in the outer layer of such skin are cellular buildup, dryness, and pigment increase. These changes, in turn, cause problems with the skin's texture, contour, and colour. The whole outer layer becomes thicker and drier because a very different type of cell is produced by the older skin. These cells tend to stick together more tenaciously and are not shed as easily as young cells. Because of this, this layer tends to build up and increase in thickness, which causes the skin to look coarse and leathery, and makes the pores appear larger than they actually are. The cells produced by the older outer layer also have less water-holding ability than those of the young undamaged outer layer, and, unless the moisture supply is increased, they tend to become dry and shrivelled. This cellular distortion causes crepey lines to appear on the skin surface, and the free edges of these dry cells tend to curl up, leading to roughness. In addition, the skin pigment increases, causing the complexion to become a shade or two darker. This would not be noticeable if the pigment distribution were even, but it usually accumulates in a patchy, irregular fashion, giving the skin a blotchy look. It may also concentrate very heavily in freckle-like areas on the hands and face—popularly called 'liver-spots'—and these extremely unattractive signs of age are permanent. (Just for the record, the liver is entirely innocent.)

As if this were not enough, a decrease in oil-gland function also occurs with age, and this further aggravates the moisture problem. Curiously, the decline is greater in women than it is in men. The final blow comes when the dry cells of the outer layer build up to the point where rough, red spots begin to appear on the skin surface. These are precursors of skin cancer, and they represent an advanced stage of deterioration. The outer layer now resembles our weather-beaten house: the paint is peeling, boards are loose, and all the trim is in terrible shape. However, if the foundation is sound, vigorous effort might still make the outside attractive again.

The aging changes that occur in the inner layer are even more spectacular, and they can profoundly affect both contour and colour tone. The supporting tissue degenerates and becomes 'lumpy.' The elastic fibres, which give the skin its stretchability, break into small pieces. Once these fibres are fragmented, their effectiveness is lost, and they are about as useful as a bunch of broken rubber bands. The weakened supporting tissue cannot do its job properly; as a result, the structure collapses, and deep wrinkles, lines, and grooves appear. Since the elastic fibres are not intact, the skin is unable to maintain its normal resiliency, and it becomes loose and sagging. The skin of the eyes and neck is much more vulnerable, and changes usually appear first in these areas, but eventually they may involve the entire face. Finally, the skin's blood vessels respond to age and damage by expanding; this causes the complexion to take on a ruddy, mottled look. In extreme cases, individual vessels become so enlarged that they appear to 'break,' forming minute red spots. These inner-layer changes, because of their location, extent, and severity, contribute much more to the actual appearance of age than do the outer-layer changes. They also have the added disadvantage of being more permanent. The skin is now like a house whose foundations have been destroyed. It has deep cracks in the walls, sags badly, and is totally unlivable. You cannot repair it; all you have is the value of the site, and you are stuck with that. The time has come to draw up plans and call in a builder, who in this particular instance would be a plastic surgeon. Hopefully, if you start taking care of your skin now, you will never find yourself in need of his services.

Regardless of how much care is given, some minor structural changes will eventually occur in every skin; no living tissue is completely immune to the aging process. Aging is predetermined by heredity and entirely beyond human control. However, the more serious of the skin's problems are caused by neglect and abuse, and these are two factors over which the individual has complete control. This point can be proven conclusively; so, if you end up looking prematurely old and wrinkled, most of the responsibility must fall on you—not your genes.

The rationale for preventive and corrective care is based on what we have just learned about the skin's two layers. Their purpose is simply to prevent or correct the structural changes that cause visible skin problems. Good preventive care essentially means good protection of both the skin surface and of the living tissue of each layer. It is worth re-emphasizing that preventive care is particularly important to the inner layer, because this is the only way to help this layer maintain its structural integrity. If you are negligent and the inner layer becomes damaged, there is absolutely no way to repair it. Preventive care is of equal importance to the outer layer, but since this layer is accessible and has a capacity for self-replacement, it is also susceptible to corrective care. In this instance it may be possible to rectify some past mistakes.

Specifically, corrective care consists of taking positive action to correct the many changes that appear in the skin's outer layer. The corrective measures we shall discuss include skin surface care, moisturization, and the control of cellular buildup. These are procedures that you're probably already acquainted with, in a general way, even if you're not doing them properly. Preventive skin care sounds much less familiar to the average person. What, you may ask, does the skin need to be protected against? The answer is your environment, a destructive force capable of causing more skin problems than almost everything else put together. Your hostile environment, which at this very moment surrounds you on all sides, is your skin's worst enemy.

THREE

ENVIRONMENTAL ENEMIES

'All the beauty in the world 'tis but skin deep, a sunblast defaceth it.'

Ralph Venning,
Orthodoxe Paradoxes

The scene is a small, brightly lit room containing two persons. One is lying completely naked on a table in the centre of the room, while the other, a man wearing a white coat, is carefully examining the naked individual's buttocks with a large magnifying glass. After completing his examination of this area, the man in the white coat turns to his subject's face, which he inspects with equal care and deliberation. Finally, he records his observations in a notebook. Waiting outside in the hall is a group of middle-aged men and women. Each is called in turn, asked to undress, and the procedure is repeated. What is going on here? Is the man in the white coat doing some kind of sex research? Is he casting a nude play, or is he just a wealthy eccentric indulging a peculiar hangup?

Wrong on all counts. He is a scientist compiling statistics on the dramatic skin changes caused by the environment. In order to have a basis for comparison, he has already visited a maternity hospital, where he examined both the buttocks and faces of a number of newborn babies. In this younger group, he found that the texture and contour of the two areas was almost exactly the same. His findings in this middle-aged group, however, are remarkably different. These mature adults have lived for many years in an environment hostile to the skin, and the least protected areas have suffered a lot of damage. In this group the skin of the buttocks wins by a tremendous margin. It has been protected by clothing throughout life and is still in excellent shape, being little different from baby skin in many instances. The facial skin, almost without exception, looks terrible.

The trouble is that we are all in the habit of leaving our handsome faces uncovered, so that they may be seen and admired, and covering our presumably less attractive areas. This leaves the face exposed to environmental attack, and the rear end, hidden from view throughout the years, always has the last laugh. Environmental exposure is foremost among the preventable causes of aging. You can judge a person's age reasonably well by looking at his face, but it would be extremely difficult to make an accurate guess if you could examine only the nonexposed skin. The error might be as much as twenty or thirty years, but you will have to take my word for this, since your opportunity to examine the buttocks of both sexes at random is probably limited. The subject of this chapter is that part of the environment which is harmful to skin and capable of causing definite physical changes in its structure. This includes sunlight, extremes of weather, and substances in the air.

The most harmful of these, by far, is sunlight. A few months of intense sun exposure can produce more aging changes than a century of normal wear. Sunlight is capable of penetrating the skin; it affects not only the surface but the living tissue of both layers. The structural changes it produces in human skin are both immediate and delayed. The immediate changes are a direct response to the irritative effects of sunlight, and the first to appear is an expansion of the inner layer's blood vessels, which changes the skin's colour to a bright red. This is followed by pigment increase and cellular buildup in the outer layer, two responses which constitute a protective mechanism designed to shield the inner layer. At this stage, these changes are temporary and will regress spontaneously if light exposure is avoided for a short period. If this is not done, and if the skin is repeatedly exposed to sunlight, the pigmentation and cellular buildup will become more persistent; even at this stage, however, the status quo can be restored with appropriate corrective measures.

The delayed changes are more serious, and appear only after a number of years. They are both permanent and cumulative, and are due to the destructive effects of light on the living tissue of both layers. The outer layer changes, which were once temporary and correctable, increase in degree and become irreversible; the final results are dark areas of accumulated pigment, rough red spots on the surface, and skin cancer. The delayed inner-layer changes are caused by severe damage to the skin's supporting tissue, elastic fibres, and blood vessels.

It is important to understand the term cumulative, because it alone can describe the time lag that characterizes the appearance of all these delayed changes. It means that the skin keeps track of the total amount of light it has received since the day of birth. Even though there are no immediate effects, each and every one of the skin's living tissues has a 'light memory,' and each additional exposure will eventually cause further structural change. The insidious thing about these delayed changes is that they finally seem to appear all at once. It's just like a charge account: you make purchases every few days and defer payment of the total bill until the end of the month. You may expose yourself to the sun only occasionally and ask the skin to 'charge it,' but in later years you will have to settle your account in full. In either situation, it usually comes as a shock to people that they have been so extravagant.

Sunlight is never beneficial to adults under any circumstances. It is required by children only because it plays a part in vitamin D metabolism. This need ceases once the bones are fully developed, and never exists at all in the child who is given a vitamin supplement. In spite of the many implied benefits of sunshine, they simply do not exist. All light exposure is harmful to the skin. There are no exceptions to this statement. The extent and severity of the permanent light-induced changes that ultimately appear are determined by three factors: (1) skin type or complexion, (2) intensity of exposure, and (3) time, or duration of the exposure. Your skin type is the only one over which you have no control. Fair skin, with a tendency to freckle, is the most susceptible to light. Darker skins are generally thicker and have more protective pigment, but even black skin is not completely immune to sun damage. Some light always gets through, and the same changes seen in fair skin will also occur in dark skin, with intense, prolonged exposure.

The amount of damage suffered by any particular skin is always proportional to its total light exposure, which is the product of the intensity multiplied by the time. You can't alter your skin type, of course, so your best chance of avoiding light damage lies in becoming thoroughly familiar with the two factors that determine total exposure. Only then can you intelligently apply yourself to the all-important task of trying to hold both these factors to an absolute minimum.

Light intensity is determined not only by the time of day and the season of the year, but by such diverse factors as latitude, topography, and weather. If you live in the northern latitudes and are in the habit of taking late afternoon walks during the winter, you are still receiving some potentially damaging light. However, if the exposure never exceeded this intensity, the cumulative effects produced over a lifetime would be very small. The situation is entirely different if you are fond of sitting on southern beaches at high noon during the summer. In addition to what is being received directly, light is also reflected from the sand and water, and it all adds up very quickly. In this situation light absorption and light damage are both proceeding at a rapid rate, and a fair-skinned person may suffer permanent changes from only a few days' exposure. The same is true of a person skiing at an elevated altitude, where the sun is not only more intense, but the snow is capable of reflecting tremendous amounts of light.

Latitude and weather are probably the two most important overall factors in determining light intensity. The southwestern part of the United States and Australia have the highest incidence of skin cancer in the world, and the older population shows the greatest amount of skin damage. This is because these two areas have a predominantly fair-skinned population, are relatively close to the equator, and have a high proportion of sunny days. The evolutionary process has not equipped persons of North-European extraction with skin that can withstand the intense sun of these areas. If your skin were the first consideration in choosing a place to live, you would pick a location far removed from the equator, with a high number of cloudy days per year. Bergen, Norway, is a specific location that has always struck me as ideal. It is picturesque, civilized, and, as far as my personal experience goes, totally devoid of sunshine. One of the local jokes is that a child born in Bergen may reach the age of seven or eight before he ever sees the sun. This is not true, of course, but the incidence of sun damage in these dark northern climes is extremely small. This explains Scandinavia's well-deserved reputation for producing good complexions.

The time spent in sunlight, or duration of exposure, is the other factor used to calculate total exposure. It is almost entirely dependent on the individual's work and recreational habits. These two things are interrelated, because sunny areas usually have a greater proportion of farmers and ranchers, and clear weather encourages outdoor sports. Active sports-enthusiasts generally look older than their lazy friends, and this is particularly true of the professionals. For a real scare, take a look at the face of a middle-aged ski instructor. If he hasn't tried to protect himself over the years, his face will probably look like a relief map of the Andes Mountains. At the other end of the occupational spectrum, I have often been struck by the fact that many entertainers have skins that look extraordinarily young. The explanation is that they not only make a greater effort to take care of their skins, but many of these people never see the light of day. The moral is that night people are usually younger looking and, if you don't happen to be a night watchman living in the Arctic or Antarctic, you must constantly be on guard against the possibility of sun damage.

There are two methods of sun protection: physical and chemical. They are just as effective as changing your residence, your job, or your hobbies, and both are a lot easier. If you protect your skin, you can go right on being a ski instructor, and even take vacations at the beach. Physical protection means mechanical shielding; it involves putting something opaque between your skin and the sun. Chemical protection means putting a substance on the skin that blocks out the damaging part of the sun's rays.

Physical protection includes staying indoors, wearing cosmetic makeup, or the use of hats, gloves, umbrellas, etc. Women have an advantage here, because makeup affords them considerable protection. This concept has gained a small foothold among the male population, but makeup on a man is still acceptable only in a limited number of social circles. As leisure time increases, people are spending more and more time in the sun, but the fashion for hats, gloves, and other physical protectants seems to be declining. One compensation for this unfortunate trend is the recent appearance of new, versatile, and highly effective products containing chemical sun-screens.

Chemical screens offer a simple method of protecting the skin against light, and they can be used with equal facility by either sex. They work by selectively blocking out the light rays that are responsible for skin damage and accelerated aging. There is a wide and confusing variety of screens available. The products themselves consist of the chemical screen plus its base, which may be a water-alcohol mixture, a lotion, a cream, an oil, or a grease. Within a very wide latitude, the type of base makes very little difference. You may use any one that suits the occasion and your own particular preference. The screen will work just as well in any of them, but you should always keep one particular point in mind. The oily and greasy bases are more water resistant; thus, they will stay on better during activities where you perspire heavily or go swimming. Remember, you can get a tremendous amount of sun just floating around in the water.

As to the screening agents themselves, we can be much more specific, provided, of course, we know what chemical screen the product contains. This brings us to the first and most important commandment of sun-screen selection. Never, never, under any circumstances, buy a product that does not have the name of the chemical screen listed on the container or label. You should always know what you're buying. The majority of products sold today tell you exactly what they contain, so there is no reason to buy a pig in a poke. Always stick with the manufacturers who are frank and above-board about their active ingredients. With chemicals such as sun screens, you have a right to know what it is you're putting on your skin. It is almost certain that eventually all manufacturers will be required to list the screening ingredient by name, but as of now they are under no obligation to do so.

Sun screens may be divided according to their efficiency and degree of protection into three groups: (1) superior, (2) good, and (3) also-rans. The following list gives the chemical names of the more important screens in each group:

Group 1—Superior
    p-aminobenzoic acid
Group 2—Good
    benzophenone derivatives
    p-aminobenzoic derivatives such as the iso-amyl and glyceryl
Group 3—Also-rans
    digalloyl trioleate
    cinoxate
    menthyl anthranilate
    homomenthyl salicylate
    triethanolamine salicylate

Although p-aminobenzoic acid is by far the best chemical sun-screen, it does have certain disadvantages. There are only a limited number of products containing it. One of the shortcomings of this particular screen is that it is poorly soluble and alcohol is needed to keep it in solution. This can make products containing p-aminobenzoic acid excessively drying for some skins. The other disadvantage is that it tends to stain fabrics a dirty brown colour. Bathing suits and sports clothes can be permanently ruined by careless application of screens containing p-aminobenzoic acid. If you are careful, however, and your aim is reasonably good, you should be able to avoid staining your clothes. If, on the other hand, you happen to be a practising nudist, there is absolutely no problem at all.

Although none of the screens in Group 2 is as potent as p-aminobenzoic acid, they do offer adequate protection under most circumstances and are perfectly suitable for routine use. They are less difficult for the cosmetic chemist to compound and are available in almost every kind of base: creams, lotions, sprays, oils, greases, etc. These screens (in Group 2 containing benzophenone or p-aminobenzoic derivatives) cover an exceptionally broad light spectrum and are used by physicians in the treatment of certain light-sensitive skin diseases. A good heavy application of a benzophenone screen will almost eliminate tanning. This is a very negative selling point as far as the public is concerned, and the benzophenones have never enjoyed the popularity they deserve. The p-aminobenzoic acid derivatives, which are also excellent screens, are found in a number of products including the Sea and Ski line.

The only disadvantage to the screens in Group 2 is that they are the most likely to cause irritations and allergies to sensitive skins. However, only a very small percentage of the population experiences these problems, and most people can use these screens year after year in complete safety.

The screens of Group 3 offer the least protection, but, on the other hand, they have none of the disadvantages of Groups 1 and 2. They come in a wide variety of non-alcoholic bases, don't stain, and practically never irritate or cause allergic reactions. The Coppertone line uses screens of the Group 3 type. They are fine for protecting against limited amounts of sun exposure. If a heavy exposure is expected, however, one of Group 1 or Group 2 screens should be used.

How can you be sure your sun screen is giving adequate protection? Obviously, it should prevent sunburn, but even then you may not be completely safe. The sun screens in all three groups block only a certain part of the sun's rays and are most effective in the 2900 to 3100 angström range. These are the rays that cause the greatest amount of sunburn, skin damage, and skin cancer. Unfortunately, the rays in the 2900 to 3100 angström range are also the ones that most strongly stimulate tanning. People want to avoid harmful effects, but they nearly always want to tan. Herein lies a dilemma and a point on which most sun-screen users are confused.

With adequate protection, it is almost impossible to acquire the extreme degree of tanning that looks so attractive and desirable on the models in sun-screen advertisements. Many dermatologists feel that any amount of tanning is bad, and that tanning always results in skin damage. It is highly probable that this view is correct. *If so, the only time you are really safe from the sun is when you are getting little or no tan.* Most fair-skinned people usually won't protect themselves to this extent, even if they know the consequences. A deep tan seems to look as good to them as a candy bar does to an overweight diabetic.

Nearly all young people are obsessed with tanning, but I didn't fully appreciate the extent of this mania until recently. Several years ago I was asked by a pharmaceutical company to help design a better sun screen. We came up with a formula that the tests showed worked extremely well—better, in fact, than anything on the market. The product was launched, and we sat back and waited for it to sweep the country. We are still waiting. It was a resounding failure, and we finally realized the reason. It worked so well that it was almost impossible for its users to get a tan. People returned from vacations at the beach or on the ski slopes looking just as pale as the day they departed. On their next vacation they used something that would let them get a tan (and, of course, some skin damage). The product was discontinued years ago, but the company still gets letters from people working on the oil rigs in Saudi Arabia begging for a bottle or two. They can't understand why such an effective product isn't still available.

Whichever brand you decide to use, always apply your sun screen liberally. Reapply after periods of heavy perspiration or swimming. This is particularly important if you happen to be in the vicinity of snow or water. If you don't tan as fast as you would like, rejoice! The screen is doing its job of protecting you against sun damage. And don't forget those other important areas not normally covered by clothing, such as the sides of the neck, hands, and lips. Even though your face is perfect, wrinkled, pigment-spotted hands and patches of mottled skin on the sides of the neck will give you away every time. You can't use regular screening products on the lips, but Chap-Stick and Sea and Ski both offer lip pomades containing one of the p-aminobenzoic acid derivatives. Dry, thickened, cracked lips aren't very appealing either.

Chemical sun screens have a tremendous future. They are already starting to appear in makeup items, including lipsticks. Although the opaque pigments and powders contained in makeup give it some screening ability, the inclusion of a chemical sun screen makes it even more effective. This type of makeup would be particularly valuable to the fair-skinned individual living in a high light-intensity area or to anyone, regardless of skin type or residence, who wanted to minimize light-induced aging changes.

It is too early to pass judgment on these products, but they appear very promising. Work is also being done on toiletries for men containing sun screens, such as after-shave lotions. There is little doubt that the use of chemical sun screens in products for both sexes will increase as people begin to realize the importance of routine light protection. The widespread use of this kind of 'skin insurance' could greatly decrease the incidence of light damage and aging changes in the general population. If the screen was not needed during the day, it wouldn't be noticed, but it would be ready and waiting if the need did arise. The wearer would also be prepared if there were any exposure of unexpected intensity or duration, and would even be spared that small amount of light encountered going back and forth to the supermarket or office.

Light protection is by far the most important part of preventive skin care. You can avoid nearly all the aging problems associated with light damage by following a simple, commonsense approach; limiting total exposure as far as possible; and using physical and chemical protectants when indicated. The greatest difficulty here is that the average person will not accept the idea of doing something today in return for intangible benefits that will not materialize until sometime in the distant future. If you start protecting your skin now, however, your reward will come a few years hence, when all your friends will look about as old as Methuselah and you yourself will have changed very little.

Before leaving this subject, it should be pointed out that a sun lamp can be just as bad for the skin as natural sunlight. These contrivances have always been popular with younger people, and quite a number of teenagers are hardened sun-lamp addicts. For many of them, the warm, soothing glow of the sun lamp seems to enhance all kinds of activities, such as studying, eating, and God-knows-what-else. The face is exposed more than any other area. This is usually done to chase away the winter pallor and give the skin a touch of colour just prior to some social excursion.

In a way, you can sympathize with the young people who have acquired this very bad habit. They don't realize the damage they are doing, and a standard bathroom light bulb will ordinarily make almost any fair-skinned person look like Bela Lugosi in one of his Dracula movies. (The count, incidentally, really knew how to lick the sun-exposure problem: spend the daylight hours in a closed coffin!) Although the dosage received from one of these electric wrinkle machines is small compared to summer sunlight, quite a total exposure time can be built up over the years. If you are practising this form of skin abuse, or some member of your family is, it should be stopped immediately.

There are products available that will darken the skin and simulate tanning, with no risk whatsoever. These are the 'quick-tans,' 'indoor tans,' or 'bronzers.' Many chemical sun-screen products now include these 'tanning' agents. A counterfeit tan can be acquired within a few hours after using one of these combinations. You can then sit proudly on the beach, looking as though you had been there half your life. While in direct sunlight, the chemical sun screen takes over, preventing sun damage and holding actual tanning to a minimum. The theory is almost perfect, but sometimes there's a hitch. For unknown reasons, the tanning chemical turns some skins a sickly orange, instead of brown. The lab people are still working on that one.

Although light is definitely the most serious, it is by no means the only environmental threat to the skin. Extremes of weather, such as humidity and temperature variations, can combine to produce a state of severe moisture depletion. This problem is most common in the winter, as it is greatly aggravated by wind and the extreme dryness of heated rooms. Taking unprotected skin out-of-doors on a cold, blustery day and then returning to a dry, overheated room will quickly lower the skin's moisture content to a critical level. Moisture depletion not only causes the skin to feel rough and dry and look unattractive, but it weakens the skin's first line of defence. In this vulnerable state, it is easily irritated by many things to which it is normally resistant, such as skin-care products and makeup. Fortunately, moisture depletion affects only the dead cells of the outer layer.

The problem can be prevented or, if it happens inadvertently, completely corrected, by the use of suitable moisturizing agents. Since these agents also have a corrective ability, moisturizers and their proper usage will be discussed in detail in one of the chapters on corrective care. Other preventive measures include the avoidance of harsh weather, keeping indoor temperatures to a comfortable minimum during the winter months, and the use of room humidifiers. Older people should be particularly careful, since their skins are much more susceptible to moisture depletion. This tendency always increases with age, due to both a loss of water-holding ability and a decline in oil-gland function.

The climate extremes that produce moisture depletion, including the modest variations in air temperatures, have little or no effect on the living tissue of the skin's two layers. Beyond this, environmental extremes of either heat or cold can act as direct skin irritants. If the exposure is unusually severe or prolonged, permanent and irreversible damage to the living cells may result. Extreme cold can cause frostbite, which often results in extensive skin damage, but frostbite is a rather rare occurrence. Heat damage is much more common, and the incidence of problems arising from this source is a great deal higher than is generally realized. Repeatedly exposing the skin to intense heat can produce changes very similar to those seen in light damage.

Strictly speaking, the weather itself is not at fault, because the temperatures of the natural environment never reach a sufficiently high level to cause significant, permanent damage. The elevated temperatures that concern us here are those exceeding the naturally occurring ones by a considerable margin; nearly all of these are man-made or artificially produced. Although heat damage may result from some specialized occupational exposure, it is more frequently self-inflicted by those who are ignorant of or misinformed about the potential hazards. Scalding water, 'facial saunas,' hot towels, and other forms of extreme heat, do absolutely no good, and they can all raise the skin temperature to dangerous levels.

Parboiling the skin is a common practice, and it constitutes a cherished part of many unenlightened routines. However, the skin is not at all like an automobile engine, and a preliminary warm-up doesn't help its performance. The body's temperature is fixed at 98·6°, and those who try to improve on nature's handiwork are just asking for trouble. All the organs, including the skin, function best at this optimum temperature, and no advantage is gained by exceeding it. There are, in addition, some frequently encountered sources of heat that also emit light, making them doubly dangerous.

The phrase 'bending over a hot stove all day' brings to mind the image of someone who is old and haggard. When you cook stand well away from the burning gas jets or glowing electric coils. The heat and light they emit may eventually catch up with you. Along this same line, it may be romantic to sit up half the night staring at the burning embers in your fireplace, but you won't *look* romantic for very long if you make a habit of roasting your face this way. Lincoln, who is always pictured studying by the fire as a boy, seems to have an extraordinary number of deep wrinkles in his later pictures. Mind you, I'm not saying sitting by the fire was entirely responsible. He did work outside during most of his early life, and later on he had some pretty knotty problems.

The aging effects of sunlight and weather have remained constant and predictable throughout the ages, but there is one environmental threat that is rapidly increasing. This is the ever-increasing concentration of dirt and chemicals in the air that surrounds us. Although worse in urban, industrialized areas, no locality on earth is entirely free of these noxious substances. Generally speaking, airborne dirt and chemicals act only as outer-layer irritants, and most of them are not capable of penetrating the skin deeply enough to damage the living tissue. Yet, although this is true of the common varieties of dirt and grime, some of the more active airborne chemicals may be capable of causing skin changes of far greater consequences. This more virulent group includes air pollutants, industrial chemicals, and the ingredients of household products, such as cleansers, sanitizers, or insecticides.

Air pollution is increasing at an alarming rate. In a sense, it is more difficult to evade than either sunlight or weather extremes. It may ultimately prove to be the most serious skin hazard of all. Under certain atmospheric conditions, pollutants may reach a level where they sting your eyes and irritate your lungs, making you acutely aware of their presence. Pollutants also attack the skin surface, but they cause no immediate discomfort. Consequently, no secretions, such as tears or mucus, are called forth to flush them away, and they continue to accumulate. The most common air pollutants are sulphur-containing compounds, which are partially converted to pure sulphuric acid on the skin surface. The destructive effects of this corrosive chemical can currently be seen in a number of industrial cities, where great quantities of exposed metal and stone have been deeply eroded. Art objects and building exteriors that would normally defy time are now disintegrating in the space of only a few years. Granted, the skin has a regenerative capacity that these objects lack, but the human skin was only designed to last for less than a century, even under ideal conditions.

The current alarm over pollution has stimulated many studies regarding its long-term effects on all the body's organs, including the skin. In the future, we hope to have more information about what air pollution actually does and how to counteract it more effectively. Some way may be found to purify our air, but this seems to be an unlikely possibility. Like the population explosion, to which it bears a casual relationship, air pollution may have already become a chain reaction beyond human control.

Physical protection of the skin is the only effective preventive measure against air pollutants. You could conceivably spend your whole life in an air-conditioned room, but placing a protective barrier on the skin surface is a much more practical solution. Since the same substances used to protect the skin against pollutants also serve as moisturizing agents, the two functions are best discussed together, and both will be covered in the section on moisturization. The removal of pollutants from the skin surface by proper cleansing is an equally important part of the approach to this problem, although cleansing comes under the heading of corrective, rather than preventive, measures.

Even less is known about the long-term effects of chemicals used in industry and those found in common household products. New ones are appearing daily, with the expressed purpose of improving some industrial process or making your home a better place in which to live. One thing is certain: none of these chemicals helps your skin in any way. The industrial worker exposed to chemicals during the course of his job has a big advantage over the consumer. For purely economic reasons, a process involving a new industrial chemical is usually researched more carefully prior to full-scale operation, and safety regulations can be strictly enforced if there is any possibility of an adverse reaction. This is not true of the myriad chemicals contained in household products. The variety and profusion of new ingredients make it almost certain that many products will be released before adequate investigative studies have been done. The chemicals contained in those products represent an unknown quantity, and many of them have not been in general use long enough to find out what they are really capable of doing to the skin. It sometimes takes years for problems to appear. When they do, there is another lag while the machinery to correct the mistake is put into motion.

The recent flap over enzyme detergents is a good example. A few years ago, all the manufacturers were breaking their necks trying to add enzymes to their products. About this time, dermatologists all over the country started seeing some very strange and persistent skin rashes. They were finally traced to these enzyme additives, and the whole thing received considerable publicity. Shortly thereafter, a flock of women appeared on television telling you how their product would get the kids' clothes clean *without* enzymes. This is just another instance of allowing a consumer product to be marketed without adequate testing, and it will happen again. For this reason, any product labelled 'new' or 'improved' should be approached cautiously and used with care. A certain amount of wariness of all household products, combined with the same measures used to combat air pollutants, will greatly increase your skin's chances for survival in this dirty, irritating world.

One good thing about household products is that their release from the container is always under the absolute control of the consumer. Unfortunately, the individual has no such control over air pollutants. As a general rule, the less exposure the skin has to foreign substances of any kind, the better off it is; and no good is done by any part of the complex mixture of airborne garbage that is constantly landing on your exterior. On the other hand, some of it may be harmful to an extent that is still largely undetermined.

The hostile environment in which you live is constantly threatening to weather and erode your skin, just as it does the earth's surface. If uncontrolled, it can line it, wrinkle it, dry it, crack it, and reduce the whole thing to rubble. But you can prevent much of this damage by protecting your skin, an option you should never fail to exercise. Why discriminate against your face? It has every right to look just as good as your derriere.

FOUR

CLEANSING—GOOD, BAD, AND INDIFFERENT

'Poverty comes from God, but not dirt.'

The Talmud

The subject of corrective care is surrounded by a vast amount of hocus-pocus and misinformation. In an era when man is routinely visiting the moon, it would seem that reliable instructions regarding the care of a few square inches of skin should be readily available, but they aren't. This situation becomes even more incredible when you consider the fact that the principles behind corrective care are all very simple and easy to understand.

This and subsequent chapters deal with solutions to the many unattractive skin problems originating in the outer layer. As we have seen, these problems are all caused by structural changes which, in time, will occur in every skin. Solving these problems obviously depends on finding ways to correct the underlying changes. To find them, however, we must first understand the significance of each underlying change. Once this is done, the specific corrective measures necessary in each case will almost suggest themselves. Let's begin by taking a closer look at an outer layer that is badly in need of some help. The following is what you might see if you were looking at a section of uncorrected facial skin under a microscope:

Starting at the skin surface, the first thing we would notice is that the uncorrected skin is covered by a dirty film. This surface film contains a variety of potential irritants that are apt to cause problems if they are allowed to build up beyond a certain level. On the average skin, we would find not only dirt, pollutants, and chemicals, but stale cosmetics and other toiletries. The remaining constituents of this film are not necessarily irritants, but, like the contents of Pandora's box, they stand ever ready to make a problem worse once the door is opened. This list includes decomposed cells, rancid oil, sweat wastes, and bacteria, all of which tend to accumulate in and clog the pores.

Just below the surface, we would find that the dead cells of the outer layer are dry and shrivelled due to moisture depletion. This causes both the skin surface to feel rough and dry, and fine crepey lines to appear due to the shrinkage of individual cells. Looking again at the outer layer, we would also find that these dead cells are greatly increased in number, since they are not being shed normally at the surface. This cellular buildup causes the whole layer to become thicker and, in turn, makes the skin look coarse, leathery, and large-pored. With cellular buildup goes a tendency to form blocked pores and blackheads, which at first would not seem compatible with the fact that the pores appear to be larger than normal. The explanation of this phenomenon is that pores are always funnel-shaped, and the surface diameter of the pore, or large end of the funnel, increases in direct proportion to the amount of cellular buildup. While enlarging the pore's outer opening, this buildup is, at the same time, constricting and blocking the narrow neck of the pore or small end of the funnel. This explains why blackheads form very readily in enlarged pores. A thicker outer layer also means more pigment and, since the distribution tends to be irregular, this gives the skin a blotchy, uneven colour.

In spite of the seemingly large number of problems presented by the uncorrected outer layer, it is easy to see that they are all directly attributable to only three underlying causes: namely, dirty surface film, moisture depletion, and thickening. Correcting these three conditions is all that is needed to completely solve the outer layer's many problems and make this part of the skin as attractive as possible. The measures that must be taken are direct and uncomplicated: the surface should be cleansed regularly and protected against further contamination, the dead cells should be moisturized, and the thickened outer layer should be thinned periodically. Since skin moisterizers also serve as protectants and the two are interchangeable in most cases, they should logically be placed under the same heading. This adjustment brings us to a final listing of the three basic skin corrective procedures: (1) cleansing, (2) moisturization and protection, and (3) thinning.

These three activities, carried out properly, are all there is to corrective skin care. Try to do more and you will 'over-treat' the skin and possibly harm it; do less, and the skin will gradually deteriorate. Almost every conceivable thing has been done to human skin at one time or another, and many completely useless procedures still have wide popular acceptance. But remember, unless whatever you do corrects one or more of the underlying changes that cause skin problems, you are wasting your time, and probably your money too!

With this as a background, we are now ready to discuss ways to correctly perform these three basic procedures, as well as the products and materials that should be used. Like cooking, gardening, or anything else, there is a right way and a wrong way, and the correct method or product must be used in each instance to get the best results.

Cleansing is the most important corrective procedure, and proper cleansing means complete removal of the dirty surface film. There are not only great individual differences in how close each person comes to this ideal, but the cleansing requirements of the sexes differ considerably because of the makeup removal problem for women. The fact that men don't have to remove heavy makeup gives them a big advantage as far as the health of the skin is concerned. Men usually cleanse very lightly, if at all, and leave varying amounts of residual dirt on the surface. Most of them merely need to cleanse more thoroughly, but a woman's problem is not this simple. If she wears makeup, she has a thicker and more tenacious surface film to remove, and this requires a lot more cleansing. Very heavy cleansing, if done improperly, can eventually cause skin irritation and structural changes. This is one reason why a woman may have a less attractive skin than her husband, who is the same age, and look much older than he does.

A woman finding herself in this predicament usually wonders why her skin looks so bad when she spends so much time and effort taking care of it. Bad cleansing habits are often the answer. Cleansing incorrectly is even worse than not cleansing at all, and many a woman would be in real trouble if she couldn't hide the results of her misdirected efforts under a heavy layer of makeup. As a first step, all bad cleansing habits must be replaced with good cleansing habits. This can be very difficult for a woman who has followed a certain routine for a number of years, but the skin can never look its best unless the right cleanser is being used, and used correctly. If we are to avoid cleansing mistakes, we must first become familiar with the various types of cleansers and how each one works.

The ideal skin cleanser should have the following characteristics: (1) removes all dirty surface film, (2) non-irritating, and (3) can itself be easily and completely removed.

There are only four types of general-purpose skin cleansers: (1) oils and greases, (2) cold creams, (3) soaps, and (4) rinsable cleansers (creams and lotions).

The first two groups of cleansers, comprising oils, greases, and cold creams, have much in common. Cold creams are, in fact, water-containing greases. Each group depends on oily or greasy substances for its cleansing action, and each is used in exactly the same way. Plain oils and greases were the first cleansers, dating back to prehistoric times; cold creams are almost as ancient.

Now, let's refer to our list of ideal cleanser characteristics. All of these oily or greasy cleansers have the advantage of being almost completely non-irritating, but they do a poor job of removing the dirty surface film. They are also very difficult to remove themselves. This means that no one using one of these cleansers ever has a completely clean skin. In addition, a film of contaminated cleanser is always left on the surface. What may have given satisfactory service in Cleopatra's time is obsolete in today's more polluted environment, and anyone using oil, grease, or cold cream should graduate to a more modern type of cleanser.

The last two groups, comprising soaps and rinsable cleansers, also have much in common. This is because the rinsable cleansers are simply creams and lotions to which a small amount of soaplike substance has been added. As a consequence, both groups cleanse in much the same way. Regular bar soaps and liquid soaps have been around for a long time, but the rinsable cleansers (also called face washes) are a relatively new development.

Let's look again at our list of ideal cleanser characteristics. Soaps and rinsable cleansers do an excellent job of removing the dirty surface film and can themselves be easily removed with water. On the other hand, soaps and soaplike substances are potential skin irritants, so all cleansers containing them are capable of causing structural changes. This is more likely to happen in cases where the cleanser remains in contact with the skin for a prolonged period, as in over-clean-

sing or incomplete removal. This is the sole disadvantage of these very efficient cleansers. It can be
circumvented by cleansing no more than is absolutely
necessary and making sure all cleanser is rinsed from
the skin once its work is done. However, even those
using the more water-soluble soaps do not always
rinse thoroughly enough to remove the last traces of
cleanser. As a rule, the skin should be rinsed in at
least two changes of fresh water at the completion of
cleansing. If the skin is rinsed by wiping with a wet
cloth, it is best to do this at least three separate times,
wringing the cloth out in fresh water each time.

Probably the most serious cleansing mistake is
made by those who use a rinsable cleanser just as they
would cold cream. No rinsing of any kind is ever
done, and the excess cream or lotion is always removed with tissue. This leaves not only dirt, but a
considerable amount of cleanser in contact with the
skin. After months or years of this, the soaplike substances in the cleanser cause cellular buildup and dryness. These changes are usually accompanied by a
marked increase in skin sensitivity and an 'oily re-
bound' due to oil-gland irritation. Since the pore
neck is already narrowed by cellular buildup, the excess oil secretion further pre-disposes the skin to
blackheads and blemishes. Anything touching the
hypersensitive skin, including water, causes discomfort, and it feels constantly parched and dry in spite of
the excess oil. Finally, the skin becomes coarse, leathery, and large-pored, with a marked tendency toward
small blackheads. Women usually react to this dilemma by repeatedly switching brands of both clean-

sers and makeup, trying to find a combination that 'agrees' with their skin, and applying progressively heavier moisturizers to counteract the dryness. It is all to no avail, because the trouble is not with the cleanser itself, but in the way it is being used. The cave woman who tried to cleanse her dirty skin with bear grease was really in better shape than the modern woman who cleanses herself into this predicament.

There are several reasons why a woman with this problem will resist any change in her cleansing habits. Under these circumstances water does make the skin feel uncomfortable, and many women never use water in any case because they believe it is bad for the skin, another ancient myth that refuses to die. Once a woman is persuaded to accept the temporary discomfort and begins rinsing with water, she is well on her way to having normal skin again. The hypersensitivity subsides after a short period of proper cleansing, the skin feels moist again, and eventually the overall appearance is much improved. Any remaining doubts about the routine use of water can be quickly dispelled by pointing out that newborn babies, who spend nine months completely immersed in water, all have perfect skins. Water is *never* harmful to the skin, under any circumstances. True, frequent contact with water causes dry and chapped skin, because even plain water will float away, and eventually remove most of the skin's moisturizers. But this need never happen. As we will see in the next chapter, the moisturizer should be replaced immediately after rinsing or any other contact with water.

In all fairness to the consumer, the people who write the label instructions for rinsable cleansers must take most of the blame for their misuse. If the label even mentions rinsing at all, it will often say 'tissue off or rinse with water,' giving the user a choice of what would appear to be two equally acceptable alternatives. The cosmetic industry employs some very high-paid personnel, and these people should be able to tell the difference between a rinsable cleanser and a cold cream. If they know the product they are trying to sell is rinsable, they should also be aware that it can irritate the skin if it is used incorrectly. Don't feel foolish if you've been a victim of this kind of cosmetic malpractice. The labels are written by people who should know more than you do but often don't. Truth will out, however, and eventually the word gets around to almost everybody. It seems that more rinsable cleansers are appearing on the market that say 'rinse off' and nothing else. Some even say 'rinse thoroughly.' This is what the label should say on all rinsable cleansers. This way, there is no equivocation and no chance for the user to take a wrong turn.

If soaps and rinsable cleansers are best for your skin, which one, specifically, should you be using? The answer depends on your age and skin type. Nearly all of us start our cleansing careers in childhood by using, or being forced to use, soap. It is by far the better cleanser. It is also easier to remove. The young skin needs this more thorough cleansing because the oil glands are more active, and the younger person is usually more active, which means a dirtier skin. The advantages offered by soap make it the cleanser of choice for this type of skin.

But soaps are also more irritating than rinsable cleansers, and this can cause problems in later years, when the skin is more sensitive and less able to hold moisture. The first indication of a problem is usually a feeling of dryness, accompanied by a slight increase in skin sensitivity. These warning signs may appear very early in those fair-skinned individuals who have been careless about protecting themselves against environmental damage. When this happens, it is time to begin the introduction of a rinsable cleanser into the routine, but the changeover should not be made all at once. It should consist of a gradual substitution of rinsable cleanser for soap, beginning with once or twice a week, and increasing in frequency until the symptoms disappear. In later years, it may become necessary to stop using soap altogether. However, a rinsable cleanser can never give your skin the deep, thorough cleansing soap can. For this reason, soap should be a part of every cleansing routine, if possible. The type of cleansing that soap offers is always beneficial to the skin, even if it is done only once a week. Many people can continue to use soap as their principal cleanser throughout life, experiencing practically no increased sensitivity or dryness. In nearly all these cases, the skin has been well cared for and protected during the early years.

Cleansers are the most technically sophisticated of all skin-care products. This partly explains the confusion surrounding them. All other skin-care products are much more elementary, and in many cases there are simple alternatives or 'home remedies' that will work just as well. Not so with skin cleansers. You have to go out and shop for them, and this means choosing one product from among dozens of competing brands. That's why it's important to know exactly what you're looking for.

There are several key points to consider when selecting either a soap or a rinsable cleanser, and they differ in each case. Let's start with the soaps:

1. *Composition*. Conventional soaps and detergents are two entirely different types of cleansers, but both are sold in bar form under the name 'soap.' Conventional soap is a single chemical entity, but there are hundreds of different detergents. The manufacturer doesn't usually tell you which the package contains, so you have to do a little sleuthing. Detergents can be spotted by certain phrases such as 'soapless,' 'nonalkaline,' 'lathers in hard water,' or 'leaves no bathtub ring.' Detergents are excellent cleansers, and oily teenage skin tolerates them very well. Most of the medicated cleansers used in the treatment of acne have detergent bases. They are also used in shampoos and, as we all know, are great for cleaning your dishes and washing your clothes. Conventional soaps, however, are milder, and they are better tolerated by the mature skin. Detergents are much more likely to disagree with dry, sensitive skin. For this reason, I always recommend that anyone past adolescence use conventional soap to cleanse the delicate skin of the face and hands.

2. *Purity*. Obviously, soap adulterated with some other substance won't clean as well as pure soap. You

will often hear soaps advertised as containing 'cream' ingredients. These superfatted soaps are simply soaps to which some waxy or greasy material, like lanolin, has been added. This type of product represents a transition between pure soaps and rinsable cleansers. Superfatted soaps don't cleanse as well as regular soaps, but they are somewhat milder, and I often recommend them as bath soaps for older people. However, the skin of the face and hands should always be cleansed with full-strength soap. If the skin won't tolerate this, I have found that it usually won't tolerate one of these transitional products either. It is always preferable to use full-strength soap if you can tolerate it. If the time comes when a change has to be made, go directly to a rinsable cleanser. Little is gained by experimenting with one of these super-fatted soaps.

3. *Additives.* The main additives found in soaps are deodorant chemicals and heavy fragrances. Both of these should be avoided, deodorants being the greater evil. The most common deodorant additive, hexa-chlorophane, was recently found to have unsuspected toxic effects. It is now hardly used in British products due to recommendations by the Committee on Safety of Medicines.

Many deodorant additives are also capable of causing inflammation of light-exposed areas. These eruptions are most common on the face and hands. I recently saw an apprehensive young lady who had developed a severe rash during her honeymoon. She suspected that her new husband had given her a galloping case of venereal disease, or something equally loathsome. Since the eruption was confined to the light-exposed areas, the diagnosis was relatively simple. The culprit, a deodorant soap, was eliminated, and domestic tranquillity was restored. Don't use these soaps on your face and hands; these areas don't need deodorizing anyway.

Fragrances are another frequent source of skin inflammations and allergies, and consequently, heavy fragrances that linger on the skin after rinsing should be avoided. In both soaps and rinsable cleansers, one current craze is for lemon. Most of this 'lemon' is synthetic, and if the past is any guide, a number of people will eventually have trouble with this chemical additive. When they do, the manufacturers will switch en masse to something like grapefruit or apple, or rose petals. Contrary to what some of the advertising seems to imply, fragrances, including lemon, don't increase cleansing power.

What specific brand of soap should be used for cleansing face and hands? If it meets all the requirements, it really doesn't make much difference. All conventional soaps are made from the same raw materials and have essentially the same physical characteristics. Once you start shopping, however, you will be surprised to find that there are really very few soaps on the market that are acceptable. I am prejudiced in favour of white, unscented bars. Many large chains of chemists have their own brands, as do supermarkets and grocery and department stores. These no-nonsense products do a good job and cause no major problems. They don't claim to be something they aren't and, best of all, they're generally inexpensive.

In other words they are safe, effective products at a fair price, almost unheard-of rarities in the skin-care business.

There is one brand of soap that deserves special mention because it is unique. This is Neutragena. It resembles the superfatted bars in that it is not 100-per cent conventional soap. It differs from them in that its mildness is due primarily to a buffering system that lowers its alkalinity. What makes Neutragena noteworthy is that it sometimes agrees with the sensitive or older skin that won't tolerate either conventional or superfatted soaps. I often recommend a trial with Neutragena as a last resort before switching to a rinsable cleanser. However, the price of this soap is horrendous, so there is no need to use it unless you have a very special kind of problem. It is surprising how well conventional, full-strength soap agrees with most people, including those who are afraid of it and haven't used it since childhood.

Selecting a rinsable cleanser is a little more complicated than selecting a soap, because there is such a great diversity among these products. To begin with, be sure you buy a genuine rinsable cleanser and not a liquid soap in disguise. Liquid soaps are usually more translucent than rinsable cleansers. If opaque, they will often have a 'pearly' look, rather than a homogeneous, creamy appearance. The only sure test is to try washing your hands with the product. Liquid soaps foam or lather, rinsable cleansers don't.

The following are the most important points to consider in selecting a rinsable cleanser:

1. *Label Information.* We have touched on the poor job done by many manufacturers in informing their customers. Read the package and label carefully before buying a rinsable cleanser. If you don't find the words 'rinse off' somewhere, don't buy it.

Another bit of dermatological misinformation that frequently accompanies rinsable cleansers (and just as often the superfatted soaps) is the claim that these products can moisturize the skin. This is impossible if the cleanser is rinsed off, as it should be. A good cleanser doesn't leave a film of moisturizer, or anything else, on the skin—just good, clean skin. Cleansing and moisturization are two separate actions. They are diametrically opposed, and you can't perform them simultaneously. It is true that rinsable cleansers are less drying than soaps, but this doesn't mean they can moisturize the skin. This distinction seems to escape many manufacturers. The harm in this kind of inaccuracy is that it may cause some people to believe they can dispense with a regular moisturizer after they have used a 'moisturizing' cleanser.

2. *Physical Form.* Free-flowing lotions are preferable to stiff, heavy creams. Lotions spread more evenly over the skin surface and are easier to rinse off. Hence, they generally do a better cleansing job.

3. *Additives.* These include medications of various kinds, antiseptics, and heavy fragrances. None of these additives have any cleansing ability, and all of them can irritate sensitive skin or cause allergies. Medications don't stay in contact with the skin long enough to do any good, so putting them in cleansers

makes no sense at all. The antiseptics are exactly the same as the deodorant chemicals used in soaps, and they cause the same problems. Unless you have acne or an infectious skin disease, your face doesn't need an antiseptic. Heavy fragrances probably are even more common in rinsable cleansers than they are in soaps. Here, too, the ubiquitous lemon is the current favourite.

If you know exactly what you're looking for, shopping for a rinsable cleanser can be a highly interesting experience. Walk up to the assistant and ask to be shown a 'nonfoaming cleansing lotion, containing no medications, antiseptics, or heavy fragrances, that says "rinse off" on the label.' You will get a look of shocked surprise, as if a visitor from outer space had walked into the store and asked to see a different shade of makeup for each of its two faces. When the girl has recovered her senses, she will duck behind the counter and start fumbling. Soon her powers of speech will return, and she will start to mumble unintelligibly. Finally, her brain will begin to function again, and her first words will be, 'I think I have one.' Given time, a chemist's or moderate-sized department store can produce one or two candidates. In smaller stores with limited stock it may be hard to find a good rinsable lotion. In this event, disregard guideline number two (the only one I consider flexible) and look for a rinsable cream.

Among the moderately priced rinsable lotions, my personal favourite is Facial Bath by Max Factor. I could name half a dozen acceptable runner-ups, but by the time you read this book, one, two, or even more of them wouldn't be available. This is a notable characteristic of the cosmetics business. With the exception of soaps, most skin-care products enjoy relatively short lives. Surprisingly, this high mortality rate is not necessarily caused by improvements in product technology or advances in the state of the art. Rather, it is another example of planned obsolescence. The cosmetic manufacturers know that novelty sells products, and they are only too happy to provide it. An old formula is changed slightly, given a new name, and launched with great fanfare. As long as it remains profitable, this flooding of the market with new products will continue. In this respect, the cosmetic business resembles the high-fashion apparel business more than it does any scientific enterprise. This is why it is better to know exactly what type of thing you are looking for when you shop for skin-care products, rather than relying on brand names.

The problem of trying to decide whether to use a soap or a rinsable cleanser may be greatly simplified in the next few years. New substances have appeared that combine the cleansing power of soaps with the mildness of rinsable cleansers. It only remains to formulate these advanced cleansers into acceptable consumer products.

Regardless of what cleanser you use, the skin should be cleansed a minimum of once a day—preferably at night, because this is the time of maximum dirt buildup. The frequency of cleansing should never exceed twice a day, even in young, active people with oily skin, and the duration should always be as brief as possible. An aged male living in the pristine environment of the woods obviously needs less cleansing than a young female who wears heavy makeup and lives in an urban area.

The water used to rinse away the cleanser should always be lukewarm, never scalding hot. Contrary to what you may have heard, it is not necessary to splash the skin with cold water when you are finished. The use of hot and cold applications has always occupied a prominent place in the folklore of skin care. It is based on two completely false assumptions: (1) that the pores open and close in response to heat and cold, and (2) that heat stimulates skin circulation. The truth is that heat cannot open the pores, nor cold close them, any more than they can open and close the nostrils, the mouth, or any other body orifice.

As for the second premise, if you need heat just to get a little blood moving through your skin, you are suffering from a circulatory collapse, and death may be minutes away. If this is the case, there's no use worrying about your skin.

As to the actual mechanics of cleansing, the skin should first be wet as thoroughly as possible with lukewarm water. The soap or rinsable cleanser should then be massaged *lightly* into the skin, using only the fingers. Be sure the cleanser is applied evenly to all areas, including the deeper skin folds. The time the cleanser is in contact with the skin should not exceed sixty to ninety seconds, and it should be rinsed off as directed above. If you feel compelled to dawdle during some part of your cleansing routine, do it when you're rinsing! Remember, it is only the effects of cleansing that are beneficial, and the cleansing itself or cleansing products are not in themselves good for the skin. Any cleansing in excess of what is needed to remove the dirty surface film is potentially harmful to the skin, so plan your cleansing routine as you would a bank robbery. Go in, get the job done, and get out!

FIVE

MOISTURIZATION, PROTECTION, AND THINNING

'Let but the moisture leave her flaccid skin. . . .'

Juvenal, *The Women*

The purpose of skin cleansing is to remove substances that are potentially harmful. But the dirty surface film that covers the skin contains other substances that are not only beneficial but vital to the skin's health. These are the skin's natural moisturizers and protectors, which are secreted by the oil glands and rise via the pores to the skin surface. Their removal represents the sole disadvantage of thorough cleansing. Unfortunately, there is no way to separate the good elements from the bad, and the whole film must be removed.

The loss of these natural moisturizers and protectors is not as tragic as it might seem. Any material, or combination of materials, that is impervious to both water and airborne contaminants will work just as well. In some instances, these substitutes work even better than the real thing.

There are only two closely related materials that are practical substitutes for the skin's natural moisturizers and protectors. These are the oils and greases. Every man-made moisturizer and protector uses one or both in varying proportions. Further refinements may be made, of course, before the product reaches the consumer. A wax may be added to alter the viscosity or texture, or the basic fatty materials may be mixed with water to form creams or lotions. This latter manoeuvre makes the product lighter in weight and decreases the oily or greasy feel.

All of the man-made products, whether light or heavy and regardless of the form in which they reach the consumer, work in exactly the same way. They do not themselves enter the skin to moisturize it. Rather, they remain on the skin's surface as a film, and moisturize the skin by slowing the evaporative water loss from the outer layer. When the film is in place, more water is received from the inner layer than is lost to the atmosphere. This results in a positive water balance, and the moisture content of the outer layer will remain at a satisfactory level as long as this action continues. The mechanism is very similar to that which keeps a dish of food moist when it is covered with a waterproof wrap during storage.

The cosmetic literature makes a great to-do about the relative merits of various moisturizers based upon their ability to penetrate the skin. But the truth is that no moisturizer penetrates the skin to any great extent, and all such claims should be disregarded. You can see for yourself that it is not only unnecessary for moisturizers to penetrate the skin, but it is actually undesirable. Think what would happen if the waxed paper or plastic bag surrounding a loaf of bread were suddenly to penetrate the crust and migrate to the centre of the loaf. The moisture would escape, and the bread would soon be as hard as a rock. (Incidentally, you will frequently hear moisturizers referred to as emollients, meaning 'to soften,' which is exactly what moisture does to skin. The two terms are synonymous, and as long as you understand what these things do it doesn't matter what you call them.)

While these oils and greases are moisturizing the skin, they also protect it by putting a physical barrier between the outer layer and the harsh, polluted environment. In this case, too, the protector shouldn't penetrate the skin and disappear from sight. It needs to be on guard at the skin surface, where the action is.

In addition to the above functions, moisturizers and protectors also act as lubricants, giving the skin better slip and a smoother feel. In the following discussion, the term 'MP film' will be used to designate a man-made product that simultaneously moisturizes, protects, and lubricates.

It is absolutely essential that some type of MP film be worn at all times. They come in a wide variety of forms and weights, starting with lotions and creams that are light enough to be worn under makeup and ending with the heavy concentrates designed for night-time use. The choice of an MP film depends not only on your age, sex, and skin condition, but on secondary factors such as the weather. (For example, a young person living in a warm climate will need a lighter film than an older person living in a cold climate.) Men generally don't use MP films of any kind, and their faces often show it in later years. The skin's requirements are the same, regardless of sex, and more men should get into the habit of using MP products. There are still only a limited number of MP films made especially for men, such as after-shave creams and lotions, but the current trend is toward more products intended strictly for masculine use. For the present, a man can always borrow his wife's night cream or concentrate, and more men might actually do this if they could be assured of absolute secrecy.

Women usually need at least two types of MP films: one for overnight use and a lighter daytime film that is also suitable as a base for applying cosmetics. This base, in addition to its MP functions, fills in surface irregularities and makes the superimposed cosmetic adhere better. The lotions and creams are most popular because they give thinner and less tacky films.

The night-time MP film is not subject to the limitations imposed by the wearing of cosmetics. Here, the skin can be fully moisturized overnight. The heavier greases and creams are generally more tenacious than the daytime products. They have to be; otherwise, most of the MP film would end up on the pillow case before morning. When the heaviness of these products passes a certain point, however, the proportionate returns begin to diminish. It is impossible to correct a neglected or damaged skin overnight by applying an inch of grease. A thin film that adheres will do the job adequately. The effectiveness of these heavier films is increased by pre-wetting the skin. This can be accomplished by covering the face for two to three minutes with a wet washcloth before the film is applied.

Following are some suggestions regarding the selection of MP films:

1. *Foreign Materials.* The light lotions and creams used as daytime MP films are frequently mixed with pigments and powders to produce coloured foundations of various shades. Avoid these. The film you wear next to your skin should never be adulterated with foreign non-MP material. The pigments and powders used to make these foundations can sometimes irritate sensitive skins, and the powders have, in addition, a drying effect. A pure MP film can help protect your skin from superimposed makeup, and this film moisturizes better if it doesn't contain powders. Coloured foundations are fine, but they should always be applied over your MP film instead of being incorporated into it.

2. *Useful Ingredients.* There are literally hundreds of oils and greases that can serve as MP ingredients. This would seem to make the subject hopelessly complicated, but it doesn't. Because all MP ingredients of similar consistency give about the same results, it really doesn't make much difference which one you use. The only important difference between the many types and brands of MP products sold is the concentration of MP ingredient, which determines whether a product is light or heavy. All oils, whether of animal, vegetable, or mineral origin, will moisturize and protect the skin to about the same degree. This applies equally well to the greases. Turtle oil, olive oil, and mineral oil show no remarkable differences; neither do lanolin, cocoa butter, and petro-

latum (better known as Vaseline).

The majority of MP products sold today contain mineral oil, petrolatum, or a combination of the two. There is no reason to pay a premium for something that doesn't offer any real advantages, but certain of the more unusual and expensive oils and greases are still advertised as having the ability to work wonders on the skin. Shark oil, mink oil, swan oil, avocado oil, and dozens of other oils and greases are touted as having extraordinary powers. This, of course, is sheer nonsense. Have you ever seen a shark with a good complexion? This business of using exotic ingredients to promote products originated in France, and for years the French were the undisputed champions, but no longer. American know-how has enabled the US to catch up with, and even surpass, the French. But the latter are fighting back gamely and have recently come up with a great one: hydrogenated halibut. It remains to be seen whether or not this fish grease will help them regain the title. The Japanese, surrounded as they are by marine life, can't be far behind.

This lack of substantial difference between MP ingredients is hard to accept at first, but it seems more logical when you consider the fact that aluminium foil, plastic wrap, and waxed paper are all equally effective in keeping food moist during storage. These different materials will also keep the food clean and protect it to the same extent against environmental contamination. If you will remember this simple analogy, you will be much less impressed the next time you hear one of these farfetched claims.

3. *Useless Ingredients.* A comprehensive list of all the useless ingredients used in MP products would circle the earth at least once, maybe twice. Among the more prominent are royal jelly, placenta extract, hormones, aloe vera, vitamins, proteins, milk, honey, egg and seaweed. These things do not belong in MP products. The same applies to what comes out of your garden, such as cucumbers, strawberries, herbs, etc. These are all great for pleasing the taste buds, but they have about as much therapeutic value as crab grass or dandelions.

It is ironic that useless ingredients nearly always raise the price of a product. This is especially true of hormones. Oestrogen and progesterone are the two most often used. There is another, pregnenolone, which is called a 'nonhormone' by its American promoters. Since pregnenolone has both the structure of a hormone and hormone-like effects on the skin, the validity—and point—of this statement seems highly questionable.

Hormones are not moisturizers in the true sense of the word. They don't work by making more water available to the dead cells of the outer layer, as do oils and greases. Instead, they change the metabolism of living tissue, causing it to expand beyond its normal size. This tissue change supposedly has a plumping effect on the skin, much the same as natural moisturization does. There is much disagreement among professionals over whether or not these hormones cause any significant improvement in the skin's appearance. Personally, I have always felt that the benefits were negligible, or, at best, extremely small.

My strong objection to hormones is not based on their lack of effectiveness, however. It's just that I'm against changing the metabolism of healthy, living tissue. Furthermore, it has never been proved to my satisfaction that the long-term application of these hormones is completely safe. All hormones used by doctors to treat internal disorders require a prescription and constant supervision while they are being taken. Skin creams with hormones have been fashionable in the US where there are no restrictions. In Britain they are not widely used: manufacturers wishing to market a cream with more than 0·004% hormones must obtain a licence from the Medicines Commission and conform to rigorous safety and manufacturing controls. By any standards, these hormones are drugs, and they should be avoided until we know a great deal more about them. Trying to plump up aging, damaged skin with hormones has always seemed to me like whipping a tired horse.

Another kind of MP ingredient that is nearly always useless is the one identified only by a trade name. There are two reasons why a manufacturer uses a trade name: either the ingredient is so commonplace he's embarrassed, or it's so complicated that he doesn't understand it himself. Trade names are often assigned out of necessity to complex chemicals or animal extracts that defy analysis. Of the many that claim to increase moisturization, I have yet to find one that actually does. Ingredients like this invariably come from small laboratories that are out to make a fast buck. An occasional sale to one of the less scrupulous cosmetic companies keeps them going. (For some reason, West Germany seems to have more than its share of these operations.) Strange as it may seem, the development of useless MP ingredients is a highly profitable business. However, there is no reason for you, the consumer, to support it. You can usually save your skin and your money, too, by avoiding ingredients with trade names. If you're going to buy junk, you should at least know what it is.

As a final bit of information on useless ingredients, don't let the term 'organic' mislead you. A precise definition of this term is anything that contains the element carbon. In reality, mineral oil and petrolatum, both of which derive from living things that grew millions of years ago (without the aid of synthetic agricultural chemicals, of course) are just as organic as anything else. Anyone using this ridiculous and meaningless pitch to sell you a product is either ignorant of the facts or pulling your leg.

4. *Humectants*. MP creams and lotions often contain extra ingredients called humectants. These substances are supposed to make the product work better, but they often have the opposite effect. Humectant is a descriptive term for smooth substances like glycerine, and small amounts are often added to improve the consistency of a cream or lotion. Humectants also act as lubricants, giving the skin improved slip and making it feel softer. They are not true moisturizers, however, and large amounts of humectants can sometimes have a drying effect. Since they have this negative feature, you should avoid any product which claims to be 'rich' in humectants.

As a result of the confusion existing between

moisturization and lubrication, two entirely different things, many MP products are still being formulated with excessive humectants. It was once assumed that anything that made the skin feel smooth also moisturized, but we now know that this is not necessarily so. True moisturizers lubricate the skin, too, but humectants have the additional ability to take up and hold moisture. They act like chemical sponges but they are stingy substances that will give up water to the skin only after they themselves are completely saturated. Because of this characteristic, humectants attract water very strongly when the air is dry, and there is always the danger that they may remove moisture from the skin at a time when it is critically needed.

It is almost impossible to make a comprehensive, up-to-date recommendation of specific brands. There are just too many MP products on the market at any given time, and the brand names change with great rapidity. Following the guidelines given above will eliminate most of the out-and-out losers, but you should also try to take a hard, realistic look at any prospective purchases.

Let me explain further what I mean by this. MP products are among the most expensive of the skin-care items, yet they are probably the least sophisticated. Their basic technology is extremely simple. Only a single action is involved: the deposit of a thin film of oil or grease on the skin surface. As a consequence, the cosmetic companies can rarely sell performance in any effective way, so they are forced to concentrate on aesthetics. The store shelves are filled with expensive products that are beautifully packaged, smooth-textured, and deliciously scented, all seeming to sink without effort into the skin. But don't let this obscure the facts of the situation. Light mineral oil (with the excess tissued off) still does just as much for the skin as the most expensive daytime base, and petrolatum is still the equal of the most expensive night cream or concentrate. Mineral oil and petrolatum won't look, smell, or feel as good, but you can buy them for a tiny fraction of the price you would pay for the cosmetic products. Even if money is no object, always remember that most of what you spend on cosmetic MP films goes for aesthetics, not performance.

Since the daytime film must be compatible with whatever type of makeup you prefer, it may take a bit of looking around to find the right one. Selecting a night-time film should be simplicity itself, but with these products, the cosmetic manufacturers seem to have gone stark, raving mad. Many of them are not only ridiculously expensive, but the companies that sell them seem to go out of their way to insult your intelligence. Much of the promotion of night-time MP films takes a gastronomic approach, and it's often hard to tell if you're in a cosmetic department or a cafeteria. Although skin can be moisturized but not fed from the outside, such phrases as 'nurtures under-nourished skin' are common. If your skin has worked up an appetite, you can surprise it with 'bio-natural extracts from France,' *ferments lactiques,*' and dozens of other yummy-sounding things. There is presently a rising sentiment in this country in favour of compulsory listing of all cosmetic ingredients by name on the label or package. The manufacturers, of course, are fighting this proposal tooth and nail. Their reasons are obvious. When the customer finds that the 'fifteen precious oils' claimed for an expensive product include such things as pecan oil, peanut oil, olive oil, safflower oil, cotton-seed oil, corn oil, etc., sales will decline, to say the least.

If you can't find what you want in a chemist's or department store, you might take the advice of a dermatologist friend of mine and try a grocery store. This gentleman believes that vegetable shortening is the finest emollient you can buy. He lives in a northern state, and keeps his whole family covered with it during the long winter.

What this all means is that the exact type of MP product is not as important as the fact that a film of some kind should be worn continually. Daytime and night-time products are made to suit almost every taste, so you need never expose your naked skin to the environment for any longer than it takes to cleanse it and do other necessary corrective procedures.

Thinning, the third and last of the basic corrective procedures, is not required by very young skin. This is because cellular buildup begins to occur only after the skin has matured. The need for thinning develops gradually as the skin ages and latent environmental damage begins to make its appearance. Since damaged skin is much more prone to cellular buildup, the need for thinning will develop earlier if environmental protection has been neglected. On the other hand, a well cared-for skin may require very little thinning throughout life.

The primary purpose of thinning is to remove excess surface cells and their contained pigment. It also opens pores blocked by cellular buildup and helps prevent the formation of whiteheads. Other outer-layer derivatives, such as the hair and nails, need to be trimmed occasionally for best appearance, and the outer part of the skin's surface is no exception. The skin's texture and contour are both improved by thinning; and the thinned skin feels smoother, appears more translucent, and has a lighter and more uniform colour tone. The pores also appear smaller after thinning, and the number of blackheads is reduced. An additional benefit is that the outer layer is more easily moisturized after the dry, hard surface cells are removed. Men thin the bearded area to some extent when they shave, and women do the same to their legs. The concept of thinning is certainly not a new one. The Roman poet Martial mentions the use of pumice and the 'polished skin' it produces. Almond meal and many other gritty materials have long been used for the same purpose.

In the beginning, young undamaged skin may be thinned simply by rubbing with a rough facecloth wet with lukewarm water. At this stage, the cloth itself will be sufficiently abrasive to remove the few excess surface cells present. The entire face and front of the neck should be gone over, using a circular motion for the forehead, chin and cheeks, and a horizontal or vertical motion for the nose, facial borders, and neck, while applying moderate pressure. This should be continued from one to two minutes, and repeated several times weekly. Thinning should always be done right after cleansing.

Older skin requires a heavier thinning than that which can be obtained with a facecloth, and something more abrasive should be worked into the routine when the small lines and enlarged pores become more persistent. The cosmetic products sold for this purpose come in two basic forms: abrasive surfaces, used alone or in conjunction with a soaplike cleanser, and abrasive particles in some kind of cleansing base. The first type includes sponges, brushes, and other specially textured surfaces, all of which operate on the same principle as the facecloth, used simply by rubbing with lukewarm water and repeated regularly. The particle type of thinner is more popular. These products are usually called 'grains' or 'scrubs,' although some carry the more descriptive term of 'abrasive cleanser.' The particles themselves are most commonly of vegetable or mineral origin, such as almond meal or pumice, but particles made of plastic have recently appeared. The cleansing base may be cold cream, rinsable cream, or some type of soap in paste, powder, or bar form (such as the venerable pumice and oatmeal bars). Products having a nonrinsable base should, of course, be avoided. The two types of thinners, surface and particle, are about equally effective in removing excess surface cells. There are great individual differences between thinning products, but by following the manufacturer's suggestions as to frequency and duration of usage the same results can be achieved with almost any one of them.

The thinners sold at cosmetic counters are not an

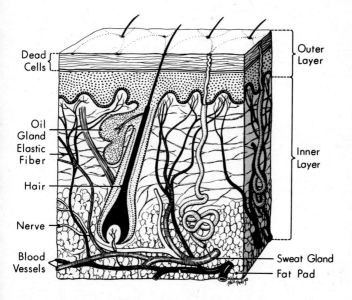

Cross-section of skin, showing outer and inner layers

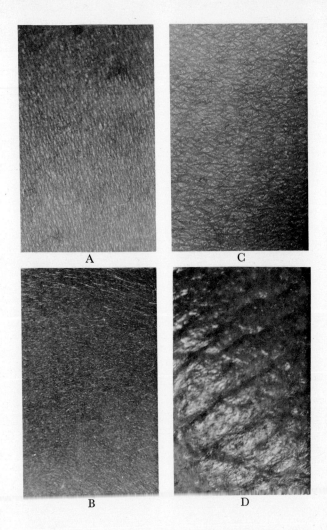

Samples of buttock skin tissue and facial skin tissue from different age groups. Photographs at the top are of buttocks; at the bottom, of faces. A and B: two-year-old girl, C and D: 49-year-old woman; E and F: 77-year-old woman; G and H: 80-year-old woman

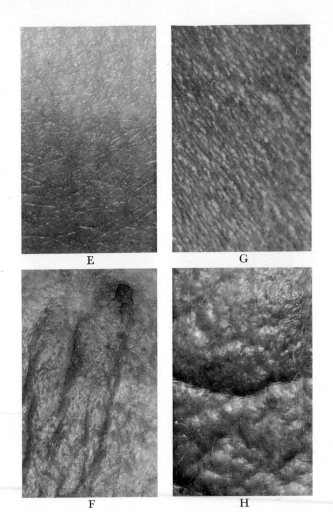

E

G

F

H

impressive lot, and all of them somehow seem a little old-fashioned. There is a good reason for this. Compared with cleansers and MP films, very little developmental work has been done on thinners. They are the neglected stepchild of the cosmetic business, and none of them is outstanding. For this reason, I don't feel that I can make any specific recommendations here. You can use the thinner your favourite cosmetic salesperson recommends and, in most cases, do just as well. Whatever she sells you, it probably won't work any better than the pumice the Roman women were using when Caesar crossed the Rubicon.

I have recently been trying another thinning method on younger skin that is prematurely lined and wrinkled. It is very simple. Grains of ordinary table salt are sprinkled on a wet facecloth and the face rubbed lightly. I emphasize lightly, because you can inadvertently remove a lot of skin if you apply too much pressure. As a matter of fact, a more extreme version of this method is used to remove tattoos, so you can see what a potent abrasive salt is. This method is definitely too rough for delicate skin, and should be used only under the direction of a physician.

The thinners we have been discussing are all abrasive in type and mechanically remove the dead surface cells. They should not be confused with chemical thinners, which work by dissolving or peeling away the cells of the outer layer (see Chapter 6). Chemical thinners are useful only in certain situations where a very specialized kind of thinning is required. They are found as ingredients in some of the skin-care aids and are also used by professionals to do deep thinning procedures, such as skin peels and chemical surgery. Chemical thinners cannot, however, replace abrasive thinners as the primary means of correcting cellular buildup.

The thinned skin always looks better, but you have to be careful with it. Having lost part of its protective outer layer, the thinned skin is extremely vulnerable to sunburn and sun damage. All skin thinned by either abrasives or chemicals needs extra sun protection. After thinning your skin, don't rush off to the beach without an umbrella or one of the better chemical sun screens.

Although the greater part of any corrective programme will be devoted to the face and front of the neck, the skins of the ears, sides of the neck, and hands also deserve attention. These exposed areas should be cleansed and covered with some type of MP film, just like the face, but thinning can be omitted. This is because the skin covering these areas is normally much thinner than that of the face, and cellular buildup has a proportionately smaller effect on its appearance.

Corrective care, which may at first sound complicated and tiresome, is really very simple and easy. All you need do is cleanse the skin regularly, replace the MP film, and thin periodically as needed. It all takes only a few minutes a day, and will pay big dividends in the form of a healthier, younger, and more attractive-looking skin.

SIX

SKIN-CARE AIDS AND MAKEUP

'Most women are not so young as they are painted.'

Sir Max Beerbohm,
A Defence of Cosmetics

Skin-care aids are a group of special-purpose products that are of interest because of the help they can give in performing corrective skin care. In addition, they may impart a pleasant sensation to the skin, offer a convenience, or produce some desirable effect that is unrelated to the correction of any structural change. These products vary tremendously, ranging from the very useful to the almost useless. Many are hybrids, and a single item may have more than one corrective effect, a situation which tends to create some confusion. The manufacturers themselves often seem to be unclear about indicating uses for their products, including what they can and cannot accomplish.

Although skin-care aids may have other desirable qualities, we are primarily interested here in their corrective abilities. The most useful skin-care aids are auxiliary cleansers and thinners; and, with the exception of a few far-out items that appear to have been conceived in Disneyland, they all fall into three distinct categories: (1) fresheners, toners, or astringents; (2) medicated or complexion lotions; (3)

masques or facials. A brief survey will quickly put these products into proper perspective and point out the areas where they can be most helpful.

Freshener, toner, and astringent are three names for basically the same product, and they all are essentially cleansing aids. The terminology used to describe these products is somewhat perplexing. Toner is a word that has absolutely no connection with what these products actually do, because they certainly don't affect the skin's tightness or tone in any way. (This quality is determined solely by the inner, not outer, layer.) The term astringent refers to certain mild thinners which were once widely used in products of this type but are rarely found in the modern versions. Since the main benefits are a clean, refreshed skin, the term freshener seems more appropriate than either toner or astringent.

The simplest fresheners consist only of an aromatic substance dissolved in water, and these have a soothing effect when applied to the skin surface. Although the sensation is admittedly pleasant, this type of freshener serves no other useful purpose. The more active fresheners contain cleansing ingredients, and this confers a corrective ability on these simple solutions.

Alcohol is by far the most important cleansing agent found in fresheners, but to take advantage of alcohol's deep cleansing action the skin must be wiped thoroughly with a saturated cloth or cotton pad. With this method, alcohol can reach and remove the bits of dirty surface film that conventional cleansers miss, including the last traces of the cleanser itself. This action makes alcoholic fresheners particularly valuable to those who are using one of the rinsable cleansers instead of soap, or for some reason cannot rinse their skins adequately. Since both dirt and leftover cleanser tend to accumulate in the pores, these fresheners are often referred to as 'pore lotions.' Finally, alcohol imparts several other minor but very desirable qualities to fresheners. It is a mild chemical thinner, making the skin feel noticeably smoother, and since alcohol evaporates faster than water, these fresheners cool and soothe the skin to a greater degree than those containing only water. (This also explains the popularity of men's after-shave lotions. These are, for all practical purposes, identical to the alcoholic fresheners used by women, except that they are never used for cleansing purposes.)

In addition to alcohol, other specialized cleansing agents are sometimes found in fresheners. These resemble soap in their mode of action, but they are milder than the soaplike substances used in regular cleansers, and small amounts may safely be left on the skin. However, they are of value only in those instances where a freshener is used as the primary cleanser. If the surface dirt is removed with soap or a rinsable cleanser just prior to using the freshener, the action of these weak cleansing agents obviously becomes superfluous.

In addition to their traditional supportive role, fresheners can at times be used by themselves to great advantage. This includes the removal of residual MP film in the morning, makeup changes during the day, and any time there is excessive oiliness. The young skin will easily tolerate alcoholic fresheners, even if used several times a day, but this frequency may eventually cause the older skin to become too dry. If this occurs, the usual method of wiping the skin with a saturated pad should be discontinued and the freshener simply patted on instead. This change in method causes most of the freshener's cleansing action to be lost, but the other, more modest benefits of alcohol are retained. Some older, sensitive skins will not tolerate even small amounts of alcohol. In these cases a switch must be made to one of the less effective water-based fresheners.

There is always the temptation to try to make a product do too much, and fresheners are frequent victims of this kind of tinkering. Of all the skin-care aids, they are the most likely to be overloaded with useless ingredients that add little or nothing to their capabilities. Everything mentioned under the heading 'Useless Ingredients' in Chapter 5 eventually seems to find its way into fresheners: vitamins, herbs, cucumber juice, etc. They are all here. However, none of them cleanses or thins to any useful degree, and they are no more successful in fresheners than they are in MP films. Maybe someday the cosmetic chemists will take pity on these poor orphans and find them a home. Despite the many claims, there are only three kinds of extra ingredients that can possibly have any real usefulness: MP ingredients, lubricants, and chemical thinners.

Only the fresheners containing alcohol will hold MP ingredients, and even then the amounts held are very small. Some fresheners are purposely formulated with more MP ingredient than they can hold. In these cases, the excess rises to the top of the freshener, where it forms a separate layer. This kind of product must be shaken vigorously in order to get the same amount of MP ingredient with each application. The main objection to the whole concept of fresheners containing MP ingredients is that only light oils can be used, and only a small amount of oil can be applied in this way. This not only gives a very marginal film, but the amount and type of film cannot be adjusted to meet different situations. The only circumstance in which one of these fresheners might be useful is during the day when a change of makeup becomes necessary, and there is no access to one of the standard MP products.

Many of the so-called moisturizers described on freshener labels are actually lubricants of the humectant type. Other nonhumectant lubricants are also used in fresheners to give the skin a soft, smooth feel, and many of these have the special quality of adhering firmly to the skin surface. They work very much like the familiar fabric softeners used in laundering clothes, and are called 'conditioners.' However, the term is often applied indiscriminately to all types of skin lubricants. The trouble with fresheners containing lubricants is that any superimposed MP film will completely nullify the lubricant's effect. On the other hand, if the MP film is omitted, there is always the danger of moisture depletion. Fresheners containing lubricants can improve the surface texture, and they are usually good makeup bases; but they should obviously be used by themselves only where there is absolutely no danger of the skin becoming dry. The young, oily skin needs little or no additional moisturization during warm weather, and lubricants generally furnish some protection. In this specific situation, a freshener of this sort can be of some value.

Fresheners with a higher than average alcohol content are frequently called astringents, although the term originally referred to certain weak acids and acid salts used as chemical thinners. Some of these acidic substances also exhibit other desirable properties to a small extent, such as bleaching and anti-bacterial activity. They were once a standard part of almost every freshener formula, but they are inefficient pore thinners, and their use has declined considerably. Astringents of the acid salt type are still alive and well, however. Even though their other effects on the skin are negligible, they do have very powerful antiperspirant properties and are now used as the principal ingredient of practically every modern deodorant. Consequently, most people are still using astringents in spite of themselves. The cosmetic chemist has wisely moved them from the face, which doesn't really need them, to the armpit, which often needs them very badly.

How do you go about selecting a suitable freshener? Well, since alcohol is the only active ingredient of any importance, and it always has an unmistakable odour, it's very easy. If you happen to be on a budget, or can't get to a store, you can make a very satisfactory freshener by mixing one part rubbing alcohol and four parts water.

Medicated lotions closely resemble fresheners, and

are used in exactly the same way. The most significant difference between the two is that medicated lotions always contain a chemical thinner. In addition, they usually have more alcohol and an antibacterial agent. Medicated lotions may be either cleanser-thinners or thinners only, depending on how they are used. As with alcoholic fresheners, the skin must be wiped with a saturated pad to get much cleansing effect.

Medicated lotions have a great deal in common with the dermatological prescriptions used in the treatment of acne and are designed for the young oily skin, which is prone to blackheads and blemishes. The chemical thinner decreases blackhead formation by clearing the pore openings, the antibacterial agent suppresses blemishes, and the higher alcohol content aids in the removal of excess oil and surface bacteria.

These products are very effective in combating the young skin's special problems, but, like all alcoholic lotions, they may cause excessive dryness or irritate older skin. This becomes a problem only with the medicated lotions that are sold to 'clarify' the mature skin. In this instance, the object is to thin the entire skin surface rather than just the pores. For this purpose, however, abrasive thinners are much more satisfactory than medicated lotions. They are also much less likely to cause dryness or irritate the mature skin. If someone tries to sell you a 'clarifying' lotion, don't buy it. Move to the next counter, or return to Chapter 5 and get yourself an abrasive thinner.

Selecting a medicated lotion is just as easy as selecting a freshener. In addition to alcohol, a medicated lotion must, by definition, contain a chemical thinner. Salicylic acid and resorcin are the safest and best. Don't buy a medicated lotion unless one of these chemical thinners is listed by name on the label.

Masques and facials have been the subject of such a variety of claims that they often seem to be products in search of the right condition. Some people credit them with powers to rejuvenate the tired and aging skin, while others feel they are no more than cosmetic security blankets, useful only as a form of occupational therapy. A realistic look at these products will show that the truth lies somewhere in between these two extremes.

Nearly all masques contain a high percentage of water, and the rapid evaporation that occurs following their application to the skin causes them to be cooling and soothing. This effect is often reinforced by some of the same aromatics used in fresheners, so the initial effect of both products is very similar. In addition, masques may have one or more corrective effects on the skin. This is because they usually contain materials capable of acting as skin cleansers. From a physical standpoint, masques may be divided into 'rinse-off' and 'peel-off' types. The 'rinse-off' masques are by far the better cleansers. Many of these contain mineral clays, which not only have the ability to absorb dirt and oil but make the dirty surface film more rinsable In other 'rinse-off' masques, the mineral clays are replaced by jelly-like substances, such as gums or proteins. These also have some degree of cleansing ability. Any of these masques may contain soap or a soaplike substance, which further boosts their cleansing potential but necessitates a thorough rinsing of the skin following their use.

As the name implies, the 'peel-off' masques are mechanically removed from the skin surface. They are based on a number of different systems, the most common ones being rubber, wax, or some type of plastic, but all of them work in exactly the same way. Like a sticky piece of tape, they remove some of the surface dirt and possibly a few dead cells from the outer layer. Technically, they are cleanser-thinners, but it is questionable whether or not they even deserve the name. Their cleansing ability is extremely low compared to the 'rinse-off' types, and the thinning action is so spotty and uneven that it is almost useless. One good thing about the 'peel-off' type of masque is that no final rising of the skin is ever necessary. This is a real advantage, because extra time is always needed to remove those small bits of masque that invariably stick to the face.

Masques cannot remove the dirty surface film as completely as regular cleansers, but they do offer a soothing, pleasant, and diverting way of supplementing them. Our interest in these products would normally end here, but certain masques offer an additional feature that is entirely unique. This is a temporary effect caused by masques that squeeze or pinch the skin as they harden. Although it corrects no basic structural change, subjecting the skin to this slight physical stress can often produce a definite improvement in its appearance. The degree of improvement is never large, and it lasts only a short while, but this 'masque effect' obviously appeals to a great many people. The effect itself is caused by expansion of the inner layer's blood vessels after the constricting masque is rinsed or peeled away. The skin immediately assumes a pinker tone, and the inner layer swells slightly as fluid escapes from the enlarged vessels. This leakage plumps up the inner layer and causes some of the smaller lines and wrinkles to disappear. If enough fluid escapes, the pores may be compressed somewhat, causing them to appear a size or two smaller than they actually are. In spite of the fact that the escaped fluid is quickly reabsorbed, taking the 'masque effect' with it, there are still those who continue to feel that these transient benefits are well worth the time and expense involved.

There are a number of other physical mechanisms that will give precisely this same effect, and some of these will be discussed in connection with the role of the professional cosmetologist. The 'masque effect' can also be produced by chemical means. Any masque that is overloaded with aromatics will give this effect to some extent, even though the masque itself is of the nonhardening variety. Small amounts of these chemicals are completely harmless to the skin, but if a high concentration is used, some may penetrate the inner layer and cause the small blood vessels to expand and leak fluid. This is due to an irritative reaction, and there is always the risk of permanent vessel injury If the skin is repeatedly abused in this manner. (The word 'mint' anywhere on the label automatically qualifies a masque for my personal blacklist.) Although masques are by far the worst, they are by no means the only offenders along this line.

Many fresheners and after-shaves contain high concentrations of aromatics and these can also cause blood vessel damage. As a rule of thumb, any masque, freshener, or after-shave that causes a prolonged cooling or tingling sensation should be assiduously avoided.

Since masques, by strict definition, are not skin-care products, there is no reason to recommend any specific one. Shopping for them is always an amusing diversion, and trying the various ones at home can be fun. Their best feature, in my opinion, is that their use always provides a few minutes' enforced relaxation. But don't go overboard while shopping for masques. There is a good one no farther away than your own refrigerator. The next time you feel the need of a facial, try the white of an egg. It compares favourably with the best you can buy, and you can scramble and eat the yolk! You don't get a bonus like this when you buy one of the cosmetic masques.

At this point, it might be profitable to briefly summarize the use of skin-care products by presenting them in chart form. Suggested day-by-day routines have been prepared for five different kinds of skin, ranging from very oily to very dry.

The normalization of problem skin does take some extra planning, but there is absolutely no reason why it should be more expensive than the care of normal skin, unless, of course, you get hooked on some of the specialized cosmetic products sold for problem skin. The cosmetic companies know a good thing when they see it, and problem skin always spells profit to them. It is standard procedure to take advantage of this situation by offering several versions of the same product, such as one kind of MP film or freshener for normal skin and another for dry (or oily) skin. In these instances, the company representatives often come equipped with 'skin computers' and other such pseudoscientific paraphernalia. These are supposed to prescribe the right combination of products needed to normalize the skin. After a few questions and a casual glance at the customer's exterior, the dial is turned, and out of these paper or plastic oracles comes the answer to skin perfection!

This sells products like crazy, but it is all totally unnecessary. Problem skin can be normalized very simply by making adjustments in the amount of cleansing done with your soap (or rinsable cleanser) and freshener. You don't need any special type of day-time or night-time MP film, thinner, medicated lotion, or masque. As can be seen from the following charts, soap is used in the majority of circumstances, but a rinsable cleanser may be needed to handle dry-skin problems. This is the only instance where more than one version of the same basic product is justified.

In these charts, the letters in the left-hand column indicate the days of the week. The time of day is abbreviated as follows: AM = morning; PM = afternoon; BT = bedtime.

The skin products are abbreviated as follows: S = soap; RC = rinsable cleanser; F = alcoholic freshener; ML = medicated lotion; MP = moisturizing and protecting film; T = thinner.

NORMAL SKIN

	AM	PM	BT
M	S—F—MP	—	S—F—MP
T	S—F—MP	—	S—T—MP
W	S—F—MP	—	S—F—MP
T	S—F—MP	—	S—F—MP
F	S—F—MP	—	S—T—MP
S	S—F—MP	—	S—F—MP
S	S—F—MP	—	S—F—MP

OILY SKIN

	AM	PM	BT
M	S—F—MP	F—MP	S—F—MP
T	S—F—MP	F—MP	S—T—MP
W	S—F—MP	F—MP	S—F—MP
T	S—F—MP	F—MP	S—F—MP
F	S—F—MP	F—MP	S—F—MP
S	S—F—MP	F—MP	S—T—MP
S	S—F—MP	F—MP	S—F—MP

VERY OILY SKIN (AND TEENAGE)

	AM	PM	BT
M	S—F—MP	F—MP	S—ML
T	S—F—MP	F—MP	S—ML
W	S—F—MP	F—MP	S—ML
T	S—F—MP	F—MP	S—ML
F	S—F—MP	F—MP	S—ML
S	S—F—MP	F—MP	S—ML
S	S—F—MP	F—MP	S—ML

DRY SKIN

	AM	PM	BT
M	RC—MP	—	RC—F—MP
T	RC—MP	—	S—T—MP
W	RC—MP	—	RC—F—MP
T	RC—MP	—	RC—F—MP
F	RC—MP	—	S—T—MP
S	RC—MP	—	RC—F—MP
S	RC—MP	—	RC—F—MP

VERY DRY SKIN

	AM	PM	BT
M	MP	—	RC—MP
T	MP	—	RC—T—MP
W	MP	—	RC—MP
T	MP	—	RC—MP
F	MP	—	RC—T—MP
S	MP	—	RC—MP
S	MP	—	RC—MP

Although makeup is used primarily for its visual effect, it can often help the appearance in other ways. Many makeup items use MP ingredients as bases, and the dyes, pigments, and powders that determine colour and finish can also act as sun screens. There are times when this extra MP film is useful, and the additional sun protection can be very important to fair skinned persons residing in high light-intensity areas. The routine use of cosmetic makeup is in no way harmful to the skin as long as it is accompanied by regular corrective care. Allergies or other adverse reactions to makeup are extremely rare today, and most of the skin problems blamed on makeup are actually due to some other cause. All of the major lines now exclude those substances that are likely to cause trouble, and the need for specially formulated makeup for the sensitive or allergy-prone skin has almost disappeared. There are still many people, of course, who cannot use one or more specific items in a line of makeup. The problem is usually caused by a minor ingredient, such as the perfume or preservative. It is easily solved by switching to a similar product in another line. Nowadays it is rarely necessary to make recommendations as to the brand of makeup one should use, and, as a corollary to this, no one particular brand is 'better' for the skin than another.

As far as the health of the skin is concerned, there are only two simple rules to follow in the selection and application of makeup. The first and most important is that all greasy makeup should be avoided. Extra cleansing is required to remove it, and this can mean a lot of additional wear on the skin. The second rule derives from the fact that all makeup contains foreign material that cannot do the skin any good, and is always a potential source of harm. The chances of irritation by one of these materials are proportional to its concentration on the skin, so you should always use the minimum amount of makeup necessary to achieve proper coverage and the desired aesthetic effect. (An almost imperceptible film of opaque material will afford good sun protection.) If your skin is given good care over the years, less makeup will be needed to cover its defects, and this greatly decreases the possibility of skin problems. Otherwise, your discrimination, taste, and pocket-book set the only limits.

The artistic merits of modern makeup and its ability to improve the appearance are beyond question. This is the one part of the cosmetic industry where the level of achievement has been uniformly high. There is an amazing variety of attractive shades and textures available and these are made even more effective by new innovations in makeup technique. In contrast to the skin-care products, you usually get what you pay for when you buy makeup.

This is a field that owes more to art than it does to science. The main importance of makeup lies in its psychological value to the user. Since small flaws will appear with age in even the best-cared-for skin, makeup continues to be just as popular as it was thousands of years ago when the first woman applied powder to her face and liked the result.

SEVEN

PROFESSIONAL SKIN CARE

'If women, continuing their present tendency to its logical goal, end by going stark naked, there will be no more poets and painters, but only dermatologists.'

H. L. Mencken, *The Smart Set*
February, 1916

A large number of people make their living selling services designed to improve your skin and, by implication, to help you look younger and more attractive. So far, we have discussed only what you yourself can do, but it may become necessary or desirable at some point to place yourself under the care of a professional. This term includes anyone who treats the skin or cares for it in any way, and it can be roughly divided into physicians and cosmetologists. This includes specialized physicians, such as dermatologists, and those beauticians who also practise cosmetology. It excludes the plastic surgeons, who will be discussed in a separate chapter. All these professionals have their abilities and their limitations, and this chapter will explore the specific areas where they can be of service.

Medical attention, administered by a dermatologist or other physician, is indispensable in two general areas involving the skin's appearance. The first is a form of preventive care, and concerns the extensive skin damage that is caused by severe acne. Eczema, psoriasis, and other inflammatory skin diseases can certainly cause you to look unattractive when they involve the exposed areas, but they don't necessarily make you look any older. These conditions often come and go by themselves and medical treatment is usually successful in controlling them during flare-ups. Furthermore, these conditions never leave scars. Acne is different. It causes deep, permanent scars. This scar tissue can have a profound effect on the skin's contour, and can continue to make a person look much older long after the acne itself has disappeared. The second area under discussion is corrective in nature. It involves the suppression or removal of various growths and pigment blotches, the stigmata of age that begin to appear only in later years.

Severe acne, if neglected, can cause extensive inner-layer scarring. After the active phase has passed, the individual pits will in time become less noticeable, but the scar tissue never completely disappears. As the skin ages, the pull of this scar tissue seems to deepen every crease and crevice. This has the effect of greatly magnifying all the small wrinkles and slightly enlarged pores. Even though the skin has had excellent care in the post-acne period, it ends up looking worn, tired, and old at a very early age.

Acne is caused by sex hormones and dietary factors, once thought to be so important, are actually a very minor consideration. It appears at a time when the whole body is undergoing a tremendous physical change, and the glands secreting sex hormones are reaching their maximum activity. The causative role of the sex glands can be confirmed by clinical observation. For example, eunuchs never have acne, and if an acne victim has his or her sex glands removed for any reason, the acne disappears immediately. Conversely, treatment with certain sex hormones can cause acne or aggravate an existing condition.

The primary acne lesion is the blackhead. The stimulating effect of the sex hormones is responsible for both excess oil secretion and thickening of the pore openings, the two conditions necessary for blackhead formation. Once a pore is completely blocked, the oil gland becomes infected and the result is a pimple or blemish. At this point, no permanent damage has been done but, if the infection is allowed to progress, it may rupture the wall of the oil gland and begin attacking the inner layer. As we have seen, any portion of this layer that is destroyed does not regenerate, and the original tissue is eventually replaced by a scar.

Since you cannot eliminate the primary cause of acne, there is no 'cure' in the usual sense. Treatment of this disease is limited to measures that suppress the infection and keep it from breaking out of the oil gland. Although good skin hygiene and medicated lotions and creams are of some help, oral antibiotics are far more effective than either. These drugs form the basis of modern acne therapy. Antibiotics are not necessarily indicated in all types of acne, but they can produce spectacular results in the deep, pitting variety. Young people will nearly always tolerate the small doses necessary to control the infection, so there is no excuse for allowing severe acne to progress to its disastrous conclusion. There are other promising developments in the field of acne therapy, but many of them are not yet fully evaluated. In older girls the use of female hormones, such as those in birth-control pills, may produce considerable improvement. These cannot be given to boys at all, and the results in girls are often unpredictable; so, for the present, anti-biotics remain the single most important group of drugs used in the control of this disorder.

The treatment of acne often puts quite a strain on the doctor–patient relationship. While the prescribed course of therapy may be very effective in preventing scars, the acne itself usually does not clear completely, and both patient and parents may at some point become unhappy with the rate of progress. This happens because those concerned don't completely understand the ultimate goals of treatment and fail to realize how much is actually being accomplished. Often the waiting and anxiety prove to be too much, and the physician will be asked if there isn't 'something else' that will clear the acne instantly and completely. The only thing that does this, of course, is castration. I have yet to find a teenager who showed any enthusiasm for this mode of therapy, even though it is unconditionally guaranteed.

There are two corrective procedures, chemical surgery and dermabrasion, that are used to treat skin pitted by acne. They are also used in the treatment of other skin problems, and the pros and cons of both will be discussed in the chapter on plastic surgery. Although either of these procedures can substantially reduce the depth of the pits, they cannot restore the skin's contour to its original state. Here, again, prevention gives better results than any attempts at correction, as it does with all inner-layer problems. Preventive measures are of the utmost importance in severe acne. A pitted skin in youth, becoming a wrinkled, large-pored skin in middle age, can be a very difficult burden to bear.

Those who neglect their skins or have drawn certain genes will need the help of a physician at a later stage of life than the acne victim. In the middle years, many skins begin to develop all sorts of extra traits that make them look considerably older. These include dark warty growths, pigment blotches, and the rough red spots that are the forerunner of skin cancer. All of these lesions are unattractive, and some are even dangerous. Heredity is the most important factor in causing the warty growths, and our old nemesis, the sun, is responsible for the pigment blotches and precancerous rough spots. A skin covered with these ugly things will make the owner look 100 years old. It is foolish to neglect them. The warty growths and pigment blotches usually remain benign, but the rough, red spots frequently become malignant. Skin cancer is every bit as serious as any other kind of cancer. Certain types of skin cancer stay localized, eating a hole in the face or gradually destroying a nose, an ear, or an eye. Other types spread rapidly to the lymph nodes and throughout the entire body. One of the most virulent malignancies known, melanoma, begins as a molelike pigment blotch.

When they are small, the warty growths can easily be removed by scraping them off the skin surface. This usually leaves no scar. The larger ones must be cut or burned off, and this does leave scars. Pigment blotches are more difficult to eradicate. If you've been careless about the sun and acquired quite a few of them, removing them all becomes a difficult, even hopeless, job. Incidentally, I have tried every bleach cream on the market and have never found one that gives satisfactory results. There is mounting evidence that the bleach creams containing mercury are dangerous, and this class of product is under investigation in the US by the Food and Drug Administration. Metallic mercury is sometimes deposited in the skin, making it a dark blue colour, or this poisonous substance may be absorbed internally. Stay away from bleaches containing mercury.

Dermatologists treat rough, red spots by a number of different methods: cutting, burning, scraping, freezing, acids, and x-ray. There is a new prescription chemical, 5-fluorouracil, which has recently come into prominence. It can be used at home, and does a beautiful job of removing very early lesions. All rough, red spots are easy to eradicate when they are still in the precancerous stage. Removal of the larger spots, or skin cancers, invariably causes some destruction of inner layer tissue. Deep, unattractive scars can be avoided by promptly getting an expert opinion on any suspicious lesion.

This brings us to the functions of the professional cosmetologist. Whether you take care of your own skin or have a professional do it for you, the basic laws of skin care don't change. Being a professional doesn't invest anyone with superhuman powers, and the skin's responsiveness is always limited to procedures that involve cleansing, thinning, and the application of MP films. Since this last function is usually a very small part of the cosmetologist's services, we can narrow it further and say that the greater part of these services consists of cleansing and thinning procedures. In addition, some cosmetologists also do certain types of minor surgery, and, as an agreeable finale, nearly all of them have a number of ingenious ways of producing the 'masque effect.'

Why go to a professional for cleansing and thinning when you can do approximately the same thing for yourself at home? The answer lies in the quality and thoroughness of professional care. You may also be able to clean your carpets and refinish your furniture, but if you can afford it, nearly any professional can do a better job. There is no denying that these services are a luxury, not a necessity. If you make the effort to take good care of yourself, you can continue to look great, even if you never set foot inside a cosmetologist's salon. But if you do indulge yourself occasionally, an hour spent in a salon is, in my opinion, a better investment than a stack of expensive cosmetic products. Even if this professional care didn't offer any significant advantages, you can't completely discount the psychological benefits of having someone take care of you. This is another reason why the professional cosmetologist will almost certainly be around for a long time to come.

The most common type of minor surgery done by cosmetologists is the removal of whiteheads, small cysts, and deeply embedded blackheads. Less common, but much more interesting is the so-called skin peel, another minor surgical procedure that is done by some of the more specialized operators. This is actually a type of deep chemical thinning, lying half-way between conventional thinning and the chemical surgery done by physicians. The penetration of the chemical determines the degree to which the skin is thinned or peeled; this, in turn, depends on the chemical used, its concentration, and the technique employed.

Many different chemicals, including enzymes, can be used to do this procedure. The skin may be left exposed or covered with tape to increase the reaction. The inflammation that accompanies the 'skin peel' varies from mild to extremely severe, and the face may look so grotesque after a deep peel that a public appearance is out of the question for some time. This procedure can also be dangerous if the operator is inept or inexperienced. If the depth of the peel is not precisely controlled, the chemical may destroy too much tissue and cause permanent disfigurement; there have also been instances where enough of the chemical was absorbed into the blood stream to produce a severe systemic reaction.

I have great reservations about the practice of allowing nonmedical personnel to do 'skin peels.' It is a very risky procedure in the wrong hands. For every competent operator in the field, there are at least two incompetent ones. Since no standard training and licensing requirements exist among the various states, there is no reliable way to judge an operator's capabilities. I would never allow a cosmetologist to do a 'skin peel' on me or a member of my family unless I had first talked to two or three satisfied clients and personally inspected the results. If your gambling spirit is strong, and you decide to have a 'skin peel,' what can you expect in the way of results? The answer is the same as with any other thinning procedure, except that the benefits are more pronounced and longer lasting.

Masques of all types are widely used by professional cosmetologists. There are, however, many other physical mechanisms that will give the 'masque effect' without actually using a masque. Nearly every cosmetologist's repertoire includes a procedure or two of this sort. The 'masque effect' is highly prized in all salons, and its chief purpose is to give the customer a glowing, more youthful skin at the moment of departure. How long this happy condition lasts is rarely a consideration at the time. Like Cinderella's coach, the skin will usually turn back into a pumpkin, or whatever it was to begin with, long before the ball is over.

Any application of extreme heat or cold, if continued for more than a brief period, will give the 'masque effect.' The methods of application range from simple hot and cold applications (hot oils, hot and cold packs, etc.) to elaborate, fitted devices that cover the entire face. Vigorous manipulation of the skin is another time-honoured method. This includes massage, slapping, and other assorted forms of traumatic physical assault. With the electrical age have come further refinements in manipulative technique, such as suction and vibrating machines. The most spectacular of all these physical stresses is the application of an electric current to the skin. The face is usually wrapped in wet bandages to increase conduction, which also succeeds, incidentally, in making the whole thing seem very dramatic. This procedure is often explained as a method of forcing moisture into the skin, and this does happen to a small extent but very inefficiently. Regardless of this or any other fanciful rationalization, the net effect of passing a current through the skin is to place stress on the small blood vessels of the inner layer and create the 'masque effect.'

There are many other things done by certain unscrupulous cosmetologists that won't help your skin. The recorded variations are infinite, and it would be impossible to even outline them here. There is usually some gadget, prop, or other exotic appliance involved, and it is often accompanied by a medicine-show pitch that matches or exceeds the theatrical qualities of the hardware. It's hard to believe that people are really taken in by some of these outlandish machines. For instance, one is an apparatus that supposedly melts solidified oil-gland secretions in the pores. Since this substance melts at approximately one degree above normal skin temperature, you can get the same results with lukewarm water. Another quack machine generates ozone gas, a sort of overweight oxygen molecule. The skin doesn't metabolize ozone, but it is germicidal, and the idea is to rid the skin of bacteria. Even if ozone did relieve your skin of a few bugs, any soap, rinsable cleanser, or alcoholic freshener could do it better. A cosmetologist can no more rejuvenate a damaged and neglected skin with

one of these machines than King Canute could hold
back the waves. The age of miracles is over, and no
one of us, particularly the dishonest cosmetologist,
can revive it.

There are outright frauds in medicine, plumbing,
and almost any other business you can name. Cosmetology is no exception, but you can't help being a
little more tolerant of the flim-flam that goes on in
this particular field. The cosmetologist's customers
invariably expect the impossible, and he is often
forced into the role of a performing magician. The
customers of doctors and plumbers are much easier to
please. If your appendectomy is successful and your
toilet flushes satisfactorily, you ask no more of these
artisans. The cosmetologist is never this fortunate.
His customers are always demanding more than
either he or science can possibly produce.

EIGHT

HEALTH, ACTIVITIES, AND ATTITUDES

'I am resolved to grow fat and look young till forty, and then slip out of the world with the first wrinkle and the reputation of five-and-twenty.'

Dryden, *The Maiden Queen*

Each skin is totally dependent on the body to which it happens to be attached, and any change in the general health can profoundly influence its appearance. The internal organs are the skin's only source of nutrients, oxygen, hormones, and other important metabolites. Anything that affects the body's manufacturing abilities or its supply of raw materials, such as internal disease or nutritional deficiency, can disrupt the steady flow of these vital substances. Conversely, disorders leading to the accumulation of excess wastes, hormones, or other toxins in the system can also have very grave consequences. Everything that has been said so far about external skin care is predicated on having a healthy, well-nourished body. To return to our analogy of the house, the exterior and foundation may be in great shape, but cutting off all the utilities will make it uninhabitable. The reverse of this, such as flooding or a backed-up sewer line, will do exactly the same thing.

The minor systemic diseases, such as acute bacterial and viral infections, usually do not cause skin problems. These conditions recur with great frequency during the average lifetime, but they are always of short duration. The diseases most likely to affect the skin have two things in common: They are chronic rather than acute, and all produce some serious change in the internal environment. The direction of this change makes little difference. Whether the skin is starved or poisoned, its condition will eventually deteriorate.

In addition to these direct effects, changes in the internal environment can alter another set of structures that are extremely important to the skin's appearance. These are fat pads that lie directly beneath the skin and separate it from the deeper muscle and bone. Their function is to cushion and support the skin, and they are almost as important as the inner layer in maintaining the skin's normal contour. Both chronic diseases and nutritional problems can cause a wasting of these pads and, unlike the very gradual inner-layer changes that accompany sun damage, a loss of fatty tissue can very quickly alter a person's entire appearance. We have all had the experience of seeing a friend who has been ill, and thinking, 'Hasn't he aged terribly!' The earliest changes in the appearance accompanying internal disease are usually due to fat-pad attrition rather than any direct effect on the skin itself. Fatty-tissue loss again differs from inner-layer damage in being easily reversible, and the pads always return to normal size when the health is restored.

These two valuable assets, a normal skin and properly robust fat pads, both depend on good general health. A sudden change in the skin's appearance is often an indication that some incipient condition is present, but you shouldn't wait for this to happen. Most health problems are difficult for the layman to anticipate, and the only sure defence against them lies in having regular medical checkups and diagnosing any abnormality in its early stages. Diseases of the circulatory system, lungs, blood, bone marrow, lymph nodes, thyroid, pancreas, adrenals, pituitary, sex glands, liver, and kidneys can all cause changes in a person's external appearance.

Although many of these internal diseases can't be cured in the usual sense most of them are susceptible to some degree of control. For example, the signs of thyroid disease, a glandular disorder that severely affects the skin and hair, are completely reversible with proper treatment. Even the most stubborn of these diseases can, in many instances, be successfully controlled with one of the new drugs that have appeared in the last two decades. Since many internal diseases are destructive in nature, the amount of irreversible damage often depends on the length of time they have gone undetected and untreated. In all cases, early diagnosis and treatment are extremely important. It is curious that people are willing to spend so much on useless cosmetic products and treatments, and so little on preventive medicine. Regular physical checkups are an absolute necessity for anyone who is truly interested in looking younger. If you haven't had a complete physical in the last twelve months, pick up the telephone *now* and make an appointment. It could be the single most important thing you ever do for your appearance.

The most technical aspects of health care are nearly always left to the physician, but nutritional problems are an exception to this rule. People are generally more opinionated on this subject and are inclined to diagnose and treat not only themselves but their friends as well. For this reason, a few additional words are necessary, even though nutritional problems are still very much within the medical sphere. The relationship between diet and general health has always been a popular topic ... almost as popular, I would guess, as those of sex, money, and religion. As a matter of fact, the health-food stores probably today outnumber the brothels, banks, and churches in some areas. The body's nutritional status can affect the skin in several different ways. Malnutrition not only has a direct effect on the skin's metabolism, but extreme variations in body weight can also affect it indirectly through a strictly physical process.

The skin requires adequate amounts of calories and vitamins to maintain its normal functions, but it does not respond in any positive way to special diets or foods. On the other hand, if these minimal nutritional requirements are not met, a number of unpleasant and unattractive things begin to happen. An inadequate caloric intake causes the skin to become dry, scaly, and inelastic, and in this condition it is much more susceptible to irritants and degenerative changes. Vitamin deficiencies can cause not only these same signs, but other more spectacular skin changes that are specific for each of the deficiency states. All of these signs are easily reversible, with a properly balanced diet and adequate vitamin intake, but borderline nutritional deficiencies still exist in a surprisingly large segment of our population. The main victims are careless eaters, the followers of diet fads, and people who just can't afford good nutrition.

It's easy to understand why the role of vitamins is so often misunderstood. The experts themselves don't know everything about them, and even minimum daily requirements have not been established with certainty in some cases. It is known, however, that the required amounts of each vitamin are extremely small, and that any excess taken into the system goes 'down the drain.' Mild vitamin deficiencies are hard to detect and, in most cases, it would take a professional dietician to tell whether or not the body's minimal daily requirements were being met. The average diet usually supplies more than enough but, if there is any reason for doubt, one of the multiple vitamin preparations should be taken regularly as 'insurance.' The reputable, honestly promoted products are not expensive, and a vitamin supplement can be taken indefinitely if the recommended dosage is not exceeded. As a final comment on the deficiency states, it has always been my impression that there are two groups of people whose skins are not only more subject to disease, but also seem to age faster than average. These are diet faddists and the chronic alcoholics. The first group is usually suffering from inadequate caloric intake, the second from multiple vitamin deficiencies.

There are always those few people who won't follow instructions, and insist on taking more than the recommended dose of vitamins. This sort of thing, if done continually, can sometimes get them into serious trouble. Massive amounts of vitamins are poisonous to the skin and hair, and vitamin intoxication can cause changes even more spectacular than those seen in the deficiency states. People who try to treat themselves with enormous doses are always surprised when their skin deteriorates and their hair starts coming out by the handful. They don't understand that vitamins are requirements, like the oxygen they breathe, and become therapeutic agents only when a deficiency exists. These same people would never think of trying to improve their health by breathing harder and faster, yet they are doing essentially the same thing when they overdose themselves with vitamins.

Before leaving this subject, I would like to stress once again the fact that there are no foods or vitamins that specifically benefit the appearance. The public is constantly bombarded with propaganda for all sorts of specially processed foods and vitamins, but the only thing these improve is the store proprietor's bank account. As long as the skin has enough calories to fuel its metabolism, the source of these calories is immaterial. Just as coal, wood, gas, or oil may be used to heat a boiler, so may a variety of foods be used to fuel your skin. Vitamins are the sparks that start these caloric fires burning; they have no effect at all on the rate of combustion. If your vitamin intake is already adequate, increasing it will no more help you look better than putting larger spark-plugs in your car will help it run faster. The metabolism always runs at its own individual rate, and you need only enough vitamins to keep it going.

Overeating has no effect on the skin, but any rapid increase in body weight can indirectly bring about some very definite structural changes. It is widely assumed that overweight people always look younger than their contemporaries, mainly because their thicker facial fat-pads tend to plump up the skin and smooth out wrinkles. Although there is an element of truth in this, it does not necessarily apply to everyone who is overweight. The final effect seems to depend not only on the amount of fat underlying the skin, but on the tone of the facial muscles and configuration of the bone structure on which everything rests. The person who runs the risk of skin damage is not the one who has been fat all his life but the one who allows a substantial weight gain to occur within some relatively short period of time after reaching maturity. The skin is literally stretched too far, and this puts a terrific strain on the inner layer's elastic fibres. The amount of damage is always proportional to the rate of weight gain, so anyone determined to become a fatso should do it very, very slowly. In some areas of the body, visible scars may be produced by this rapid stretching of the skin. These are seen most frequently on the upper thighs and stomach, and are euphemistically termed 'stretch marks.' Since the facial skin is more lax, it is never affected this severely, and the damage usually isn't apparent until after the person starts to lose weight. When this happens, the skin tends to sag and hang in folds, and the loss of tone becomes obvious. The only way to remedy this situation is to get fat again and stay fat, but this puts a strain on the heart and other organs and will statistically shorten the average life span by a number of years. There may be one consolation, however, if a person elects to follow this particular course. After the fatal heart attack or stroke, when family and friends come to pay their last respects, they will all agree on how young the corpse looks!

Very well and good, you may say, but you have been having regular checkups for a number of years and are in magnificent health. You also eat a sensible diet, take a daily vitamin supplement, and your weight is not only within normal limits, but has changed very little since adolescence. You certainly don't expect to live forever but would like to retard the body's aging processes a little. Can medical science offer any help along these lines? The answer is negative at present, but there is one clue as to how this might be accomplished in the future.

From the ancient alchemists onward, youth potions have had a popular appeal second only to the changing of lead into gold, and every conceivable substance has been tried a dozen times over. There are still reports of medical wizards living in remote corners of the world who specialize in rejuvenating the rich and famous with things like animal extracts, but this sort of humbug has little or no scientific basis. In fact, you could mince, distil, and inject the entire population of the London Zoo without the slightest effect on aging. The results achieved with exotic plant extracts, various chemicals, and most hormones are similarly disappointing. But, as an official of the Toilet Preparations Federation has pointed out, in Britain all claims made for 'youth potions' are severely restricted by the Trade Descriptions Act.

Certain types of potions seems to have an ethnic popularity. The Slavs, for instance, are particularly fond of procaine, and preparations coming out of Central Europe often list this drug as the active ingredient. Procaine is widely used as a local anaesthetic for skin surgery, and since the new plastic syringes tend to come apart under pressure, I inhale or swallow a considerable amount of it every day. This has been going on for a number of years, and as far as I can tell, the stuff hasn't helped my appearance one bit. There have been several hints in the medical literature recently that hormones of the types used in birth-control pills may retard some aspects of aging, but at present most of the controversy concerning these drug centres on their undesirable side effects. However, if a safe, effective fountain of youth is ever found, it will probably be an internally administered hormone or cellular metabolite.

Finally, there are a number of other less well-defined factors, not related to the general health or state of nutrition, which are also thought to have a strong influence on the aging processes. These are a person's physical and mental habits, or activities and attitudes. Most authorities agree that severe physical or mental stress can definitely cause bodily changes, and we know that the amount of stress each person encounters in his daily life is determined to a large extent by his activities and attitudes. The study of these stresses and their effects on the body lies for the most part within the realms of physical and psycho-somatic medicine. These are areas rich in theory and opinion but often poor in proven scientific fact, and some of the observed results are hard to explain. We have all had the experience of knowing someone who seemed to age very rapidly after undergoing a severe stress of some kind. Much physical and mental stress is caused by circumstances that are beyond human control, but many of the routine stresses to which we are all exposed each day can be anticipated and avoided. These stresses often have a cumulative effect, and nearly every life pattern contains something that can be rearranged or eliminated so as to reduce stress to a mimimum.

Is there any real relationship between aging and a person's activities and attitudes? This cannot be answered with any degree of assurance at this time, but I personally believe there is a correlation and that a certain life pattern frequently goes with a younger appearance. I have examined a tremendous amount of skin during my many years as a dermatologist and have always made an effort to investigate the personal lives and habits of those patients who seem to look much younger or much older than their contemporaries. From this, I have tried to evolve a profile of the younger looking person. I would like to present this, not as a scientific study, but as a series of strictly personal impressions. The following are some of the more conspicuous things that many well-preserved people seem to have in common: (1) married, with fewer children than average, (2) regular habits of rest and exercise, and (3) more interests and hobbies.

It is a statistical fact that married people live longer. Connubial living, in some mysterious way, seems to help preserve the human machinery. On the other hand, the fruits of marital union, in excess, do the opposite, and the parents of a large brood often age quite rapidly. There is an old saying to the effect that women are 'worn out' by child-bearing, but there are two very good reasons for doubting the truth of this old wives' tale. We now know that the pregnant state is actually beneficial to women in many ways, and the fathers seem to be equally affected by a large litter. Therefore, it is probably not the bearing of children that adds the wrinkles, but the physical and mental stresses caused by raising them. Granted, the mothers are more directly concerned with the care of the children, but the fathers have equal or greater problems in trying to provide for them. Exceptions to this situation are found among the very wealthy, who seem to have children by the dozen with no ill effects. Plentiful servants and guaranteed financial security obviously do much to protect these fortunate people from the hazards of procreation. Limiting the number of children would seem to be attractive to the average person on several counts. There would not only be the satisfaction derived from a negative contribution to the population problem, but it might also help to preserve the potential parents.

There is absolutely no doubt that regular rest and exercise are important to your appearance. These good habits are not acquired automatically, and developing them usually takes some planning and effort. Inadequate rest can lead to chronic fatigue, the aging effects of which are familiar to everyone. No one can look his best without the proper amount of sleep. This means regular sleep, not ten hours one night and five the next. Even if all the other personal habits are exemplary, those who are careless about scheduling the same amount of sleep every night will fade much earlier in life than those who follow a set routine. It is also desirable to plan several five-to-ten-minute periods of relaxation during the day. To do this, lie down, or lean back in a chair and close your eyes. Let your body go limp, and try to think of something other than your immediate problems.

The body also needs some form of regular exercise to stay in top condition, but the amount and type of exercise needed varies from person to person. Here, too, regularity is very important. Unlike rest, exercise can be overdone, and improper exercise does more harm than good. You should never under any circumstances, subject your body to violent bursts of activity for which it is unprepared. This is often called the 'weekend athletic' syndrome. Punishing yourself in this manner won't help your looks, but it may end all your aging problems by giving you a fatal coronary. Irregular habits of rest and exercise cause physical stress, and this always increases the susceptibility to mental stress. The person who rests and exercises sensibly is more immune to all forms of stress, and usually shows it.

I have also found that younger-looking people tend to have interests and hobbies of the kinds that offer a challenge. These all involve some form of active mental exercise, which is good, and this can displace mental stress, which is bad. The mind is being used in both instances, but the psychosomatic effects are entirely different. Doing a crossword puzzle or reading a difficult book may require some hard mental exertion, but it is actually relaxing in many ways, and the systemic effects are definitely beneficial. An equal amount of mental energy may be devoted to worrying about the unpaid bills, but this only creates tensions. Completely passive mental activity, such as watching the sunset or listening to music, doesn't count either way. In my experience, the youngest-looking people have always been those who were eager to learn about new and unfamiliar subjects or were always deeply involved in some interesting project. When they had mastered any particular subject to the best of their abilities, or exhausted its possibilities, they would move on to something else. This involvement might be anything from taking a bridge course at the YMCA to working with local charitable or political groups. Almost all the experts agree that mental inactivity is often a prelude to physical deterioration. They also agree that pushing the mind to the limits of its ability will definitely help preserve the overall health and appearance. Without doubt, mental exertion is one of the most important keys to the secret of looking younger. Stress is impossible to avoid altogether, even in the best arranged life, and some of it must be accepted as part of doing a job or running a home. However, it always seems to have the least effect on those who cultivate an active and inquiring mind.

NINE

LAST RESORTS

'My skin hangs about me like an old lady's loose gown.'
Shakespeare, *Macbeth*

Our study of tired and aging skin concludes with a discussion of the surgical techniques designed to restore it to a more youthful state. This brings us full circle, for the history of plastic surgery also begins with the ancient Egyptians, who first tried to eliminate wrinkles by stuffing the mouths of the dead with cotton prior to mummification. It is entirely possible that the same fellow who concocted the facial masque also had a hand in this pioneering development. Perhaps the masque was not selling as well as expected, and he finally came to the conclusion that the mortuary business not only offered more security but also much less chance of a dissatisfied customer.

The modern plastic surgeon, the spiritual heir of these ancient morticians, is to me the most interesting of all medical specialists. In addition to being a highly competent technician, he must also have a certain amount of artistic ability if he is to perform his work with any degree of distinction. People possessing both practical and creative talents sometimes seem to have difficulty reconciling the two, and plastic surgeons, who usually differ temperamentally from other physicians, are no exception. They all have a tendency to worry about their image and often seem acutely embarrassed by the cosmetic aspects of their work, which they are afraid will seem frivolous to their medical colleagues. These apprehensions are groundless, of course, but a large segment of the public still seems to be unaware that the field of plastic surgery consists of anything more than an endless series of cosmetic operations on ugly old faces and undersized breasts.

The plastic surgeon has two things to offer the individual with aging and damaged skin. The first is chemical surgery, which is aimed primarily at improving the skin's texture, and the better known face-lift, which corrects contour problems. To achieve the best possible results it may be necessary to do both of these operations on the same skin, either in whole or in part.

In chemical surgery, a caustic is used to destroy the entire outer layer and part of the adjoining inner layer. This eliminates not only the old layer itself, which is thickened and large-pored; but it also gets rid of all the ugly things that are contained within or attached to it, such as the familiar warty growths, pigment blotches, and rough spots. The removal of a portion of the inner layer stimulates the growth of the new tissue in this area and helps promote a partial rebuilding of the skin. At the conclusion of this procedure, the patient has no outer layer at all, about two-thirds of the inner layer, and a face that is eminently suitable for a Halloween party. The final results, however, may be truly astonishing, with as much as a decade or two seeming to disappear from the face. A new outer layer, which regrows completely from the hair root and oil-gland linings, is responsible for the greater part of this very striking improvement. The skin is extremely smooth and small-pored, and is rid of all the unattractive baggage it had accumulated over the years. The healed inner layer is somewhat thicker than before, as well as being firmer and more resilient. This new inner-layer tissue has the effect of plumping up the skin and erasing many small lines and wrinkles. Although the contour changes are of a lesser magnitude than the texture changes conferred by a brand-new outer layer, they do make a substantial contribution to the overall improvement.

The maximum benefits of chemical surgery may not be fully realized for three to six months. The entire face or neck must be treated initially to avoid contrasting areas, but local 'touch-ups' can be done later if necessary. Chemical surgery is also used to treat skin pitted by acne, and although the results are gratifying in most cases, they are far less dramatic than those obtained in the treatment of aging skin.

The advantages of chemical surgery sound almost too good to be true. It makes you wonder why you can't just forget about your skin and have this operation done at the first signs of age. So far, only the benefits of chemical surgery have been mentioned, but there are some definite drawbacks and, as with any operation, a chance of complications. There is really not as much pain and discomfort associated with this procedure as you might expect, but the caustic does cause an intense and unsightly inflammation that precludes any social engagements for quite some time. The most important drawback, in my opinion, is that the skin never looks entirely normal again. The new skin often has a slightly artificial look about it, as though it might be of some synthetic material. This is due to the fact that the regenerated portion of the inner layer consists entirely of scar tissue and therefore lacks the tone and pliability of the original article. It is also much less durable than normal tissue. This means that the new skin will not last the better part of a lifetime, like the old one, but will relapse completely in one to ten years. The exact time depends to a large extent on the care given the new skin, but eventually the operation will have to be repeated if the effect is to be maintained.

In addition, certain unexpected complications may result from chemical surgery, even in highly skilled hands. The most common is the formation of excess pigment, which may be several times the amount that was present originally. The exact cause of this complication is unknown, but a particularly intense reaction to the caustic and prematurely exposing the skin to strong sunlight both have been cited as contributing factors. The reverse of this can occur as well, and sometimes the original skin pigment fails to return altogether. In other cases, the skin is left with a very obvious ruddy tint, also unattractive, due to an abnormal enlargement of the small blood vessels. Any one of these distressing complications can be a cosmetic disaster and create some very difficult problems for the person involved. Lastly, there is always the possibility of scarring and disfigurement, due to error on the part of the surgeon, or some other unforeseen mishap.

There is an alternative to chemical surgery, known as dermabrasion, where the tissue is removed with a rotating wire brush or steel burr rather than a caustic. The two methods give equivalent results, and can be used interchangeably in the treatment of both acne pits and aging skin. Statistically speaking, dermabrasion seems to be preferred in the first instance, and chemical surgery in the second. There are other more technical differences between these two procedures that may affect the decision as to which should be used in each particular case, but a skilled operator can achieve excellent results with either one. If a person is willing to accept the discomfort, inconvenience, and risk, both of these operations can offer a temporary solution to the skin's aging problems and a much younger appearance.

The face-lift is a real honest-to-goodness cutting and stitching type of surgery, and both the indications and final results are quite different from those of chemical surgery and dermabrasion. The face that benefits most from this operation is one with a severe contour problem, with deep lines; wrinkles; and loose, sagging skin that hangs in folds. Although sun damage plays a major role in causing these defects, other contributing factors are usually found in those cases where the furrows, lines, and skin folds are especially pronounced. Of these, the pull of the facial muscles and a loss of fat pads are the two most important. The deeper and more noticeable skin lines are always found about the eyes, mouth, and forehead, which are the areas most used in forming facial expressions. In particularly animated individuals, the depth of these lines can be greatly increased by muscle pull, which further stretches an already tired and inelastic skin. A loss of the supporting fat pads not only increases wrinkling, but it also accounts for much of the looseness and folding found in older skin. As we have seen, these pads may temporarily diminish in size due to disease or nutritional problems. However, they often undergo a gradual atrophy with age, even in healthy and well-nourished individuals.

Originally, a face-lift consisted simply of making an incision in the skin, stretching it tight, cutting off the excess skin, and sewing the ends back together. However, the pull of the facial muscles on the stretched and damaged skin soon caused the face to relapse to its preoperative state. The modern method includes re-attachment of the facial muscles to minimize their pull, a practice that greatly extends the life of this operation. Unfortunately, it also causes a loss of facial expression that is directly proportional to the degree of face-lift, so it is theoretically possible to end up looking very much younger but have a face that is almost completely expressionless. The surgeon always attempts to achieve an exact balance between those two elements, and doing this properly requires both a high level of technical competence and a well-developed aesthetic sense. A local anaesthetic is often used, so that the patient, with the aid of a mirror, can observe the operation's progress and discuss it with the surgeon. In this way, the personal desires of the patient can be better expressed, and there is much less chance of being disappointed with the final results.

There are also limited corrective procedures available for specific problem areas in cases where a major face-lift is not indicated. A 'mini-lift' can be done to correct a deeply lined forehead, baggy eyelids, or a sagging, wrinkled neck. The forehead and upper lip usually respond less well to a face-lift than other areas, and can be given supplementary treatment, if necessary, with chemical surgery or dermabrasion.

A major face-lift can be expected to last, on the average, from three to five years. The best and most enduring results are obtained in those cases where the skin itself is comparatively undamaged and most of the contour changes are caused by muscle pull or a loss of fat pads. Where extensive inner layer damage is present, the poor resiliency of the stretched skin sometimes causes the face to take on a masklike appearance following the operation. This is another reason for always practising good preventive skin care. If it ever becomes necessary for you to have this operation, then at least there will be something left for the surgeon to lift.

The treatment of lines and wrinkles by the injection of silicone fluid is another plastic procedure that has received considerable publicity. It has been much more widely used in America than in Britain where only a small number of plastic surgeons make use of it to eradicate facial wrinkles and frownlines. Recently in the US where its unauthorized use was fairly widespread, a reappraisal has been carried out by the Food and Drug Administration. The theory behind its use is simple: The fluid is injected directly into the skin to expand and firm the inner layer, and is also introduced beneath the skin to replace the lost fat pads. The method is quick, easy to do, and relatively painless. Since the results are excellent, it would otherwise be the treatment of choice for isolated lines and furrows, but silicone injections are potentially dangerous. The fluid doesn't always stay where it's put but has a tendency to migrate away from the injection site. It can even enter the general circulation, and droplets of silicone fluid have been found in the brain, liver, and other vital organs. In view of this, and the distinct possibility that there may be other long-term side effects which are unknown at this time, these injections are definitely contra-indicated. The theory is a good one, however, and perhaps a completely safe injection technique will be developed at some future date.

The future, in fact, may bring all sorts of amazing things to the field of plastic surgery. It may be possible someday to draw on skin banks for the total replacement of aging skin, or we may even see the development of an entirely synthetic skin that would require no maintenance and never show damage or age. With either of these things, a person might conceivably be able to look almost any age at all. This could be a real boon to the older generation, which at this point would seem to need all the help it can get. The ever-widening gap between the extremes of age in our society seems, at times, to have spawned two separate and distinct races, the young and the old. As

the number of young people in our population increases, the older generation is finding itself more and
more an alien minority in a world dominated by its
youth. The breach between those two groups is obviously growing deeper all the time, communications
are breaking down, and any step toward a reconcilia-
tion would be welcomed by both sides. It is tempting
to think that narrowing the physical differences between the two might solve part of the problem, but
putting a younger face on an older person, by itself,
would accomplish very little. Young ideas, or at least
more flexible ones, are much more important than a
young face. In the final analysis, it is not appearance,
but ways of thinking, that represent the ultimate barrier to a man's search for rejuvenation.

TEN

THE HAIR, HANDS, AND NAILS

'A fine head of hair adds beauty to a good face, and terror to an ugly one.'

Lycurgus,
Plutarch's *Lives*

A full, healthy head of hair is indispensable as an accessory to a well-cared-for skin. The hair and skin are mutually complementary, and if one is allowed to deteriorate, the other also seems to suffer. In judging a person's overall appearance, we are likely to assign a disproportionately high value to the hair. There may be other explanations for this tendency, but the most likely one is that we are all conditioned to associate healthy, luxuriant hair with a young skin. In addition, this curious appendage has a quality or mystique all its own, and a woman with damaged, thinning hair, or a bald man, will automatically look many years older. This is always the first impression, even though the skin itself is in excellent condition, Nothing alarms the average person more, or has a greater psychological impact, than the sudden onset of hair loss, The quantity of hair a person has, however, is not the only consideration. The quality or health of each individual hair is also very important, and the object of the game is not only to keep as much hair as you can but to have it in the best possible condition.

The thickness or quantity of hair is always the most important consideration. There are four general causes for a decrease in quantity or hair loss: (1) systemic, (2) scalp disease, (3) heredity, and (4) mechanical trauma.

Reaction to drugs and internal diseases are the most frequently encountered systemic causes of hair loss. Either of these situations may cause widespread hair loss, or even total baldness. For instance, a thinning head of hair is often the first sign of vitamin A intoxication. Unusual reactions to hormones, and a host of other drugs, can also cause hair loss, even though the recommended dosages are strictly observed. Among the internal diseases, glandular disturbances account for most of the hair-loss problems seen in physicians' offices. Abnormal thyroid function is the chief culprit. The thyroid status should be the first thing checked in any case of progressive hair loss where no medication is being taken and the cause is not immediately apparent. Women normally experience a number of special hormonal changes and adjustments during their lives that are in some instances associated with hair loss. The hair often becomes much thinner at the time of menopause, and a rather heavy loss can occur three to six months after childbirth. While the menopausal loss is usually permanent, the loss due to childbirth is not, and the hair will nearly always return spontaneously to its original thickness.

More patients are being seen by physicians these days with another type of hair loss where the cause, although undoubtedly systemic, cannot be traced to any definite source. There is always a history that the hair, for no apparent reason, has suddenly become extremely thin. The picture very closely mimics that seen in thyroid disease, but all of the tests are negative. When the doctor cannot come up with a reasonable explanation, the patient often feels obliged to invent one and becomes convinced that the problem is being caused by something like pesticides or radioactive fallout. The incidence of this puzzling affliction appears to be on the increase, but I believe this is not really the case. The explanation is simply that more people are seeking professional help. For lack of a better name, this type of hair loss is often referred to as 'ideopathic,' which is Greek for 'I don't know, either.' The hair in these cases may remain permanently thin, or it may, in time, return to its original thickness, even though there has been absolutely no change in the person's habits or physical condition. Nutritional deficiencies, often suspected in these 'ideopathic' cases, are rarely a cause of hair loss. As a matter of fact, a person will usually starve to death long before any appreciable quantity of hair comes out. All of these systemic problems must be investigated by a physician. The abnormality may be susceptible to complete control, as thyroid disease usually is, or assurance that the problem is self limited and will eventually correct itself may be all that is needed.

The scalp diseases that are associated with hair loss include not only the common bacterial and fungal infections, but a number of inflammatory conditions of unknown origin. These scalp inflammations are all less well understood than the infections and are generally much more difficult to treat. The two most common, localized baldness and dandruff, deserve special mention. Localized baldness (or *alopecia areata*) appears as round or irregularly shaped hairless areas that can occur on any part of the scalp. The disease may be limited to one pea-sized spot, or there may be multiple areas that rapidly enlarge and coalesce until the scalp is completely bald. The cause of this distressing malady is unknown, although various toxic and psychosomatic factors have been implicated. It is by no means a rare condition, and many a person has become highly alarmed on finding, or having a barber or hairdresser find, a completely hairless area on some part of the scalp. Fortunately, the hair will regrow spontaneously in the majority of cases, although this may take quite some time. Localized baldness is often confused by the public with other types of hair loss, and victims of this condition often fall prey to one of the so-called hair experts who advertise their powers in the newspapers. The 'expert' then proceeds to exploit the initial panic by selling the balding man or woman a course of expensive treatments. When the hair finally regrows of its own accord, the therapist receives some undeserved credit.

Dandruff is by far the most common scalp disease associated with hair loss. Actually, the disease itself does not affect the hair roots, and so it is not directly responsible for the thinning head of hair that usually accompanies it. The explanation lies in the fact that dandruff itches, sometimes severely, and the itch is always scratched. The fingernails can be deadly weapons as far as the hairs are concerned, and large numbers of them can be broken off close to the scalp by vigorous scratching. The scalp itself is always cut and nicked in the process, and the development of a secondary bacterial infection can further accelerate the loss.

Nearly all the bacterial and fungal infections that attack the scalp can be completely eradicated by appropriate medical treatment. However, most of the scalp inflammations are not curable in the sense that some course of therapy will permanently eliminate them. In dandruff, for instance, the sufferer must be satisfied with achieving control of the process and a suppression of the annoying symptoms. Technically, dandruff is a skin disease, a distant cousin of eczema and psoriasis. The more severe forms require treatment by a physician. The average case, however, can be controlled by a non-prescription medicated shampoo. There are many on the market in Britain (Vosene and Loxene are among the most popular). Medicated shampoos often contain different active ingredients—an important point since you may need to change shampoos somewhere along the line. Every dandruff shampoo works well at first, but its effectiveness usually decreases after you have used it for a while. When your dandruff shampoo stops working switch to one with a different active ingredient. This way, you'll be able to get the dandruff under control again—for a while.

The hereditary type of hair loss may progress to complete baldness in men, but it never affects women to this extent. This is because men have something in their systems women don't: a high level of male hormone. If the main source of this is removed early in life by castration, a man can never become completely bald. (When you consider the effects of the male sex glands on both hair and adolescent acne, they would seem to be more of a liability than an asset, at least as far as the masculine appearance is concerned.) The fact that male homosexuals become just as bald as their heterosexual counterparts has been cited as one proof that homosexuals have no hormonal abnormality. Sexual preferences, it would seem, have a mental rather than a glandular determination.

I often find that balding men are reluctant to accept heredity as the cause of their problem and, like the victims of 'ideopathic' hair loss, constantly search for another explanation. One of my good friends remains convinced to this day that his own baldness resulted from the use of transmission grease from his tank as a substitute hair dressing during World War II. I have been unable to dissuade him of this notion, and I am not so sure I should keep trying. Defective genes of any kind are apparently a sensitive subject, even though the trait they carry is a completely harmless one, like baldness.

The pattern of male hereditary hair loss is very characteristic, being localized at onset to the front hairline and crown. This diagnosis is much more difficult to make in women, because the loss is never as distinct or as well localized, and the pattern is often indistinguishable from that seen in systemic hair loss. The most important thing to remember about hereditary hair loss is that it doesn't always continue to progress at a constant rate in either sex. The young man who is losing his hair very rapidly may find that the loss will eventually slow down or stop altogether. Being aware of this fact can be a great comfort to the man or woman who obviously would become completely bald if the initial rate of loss were to continue indefinitely.

The final cause of hair loss is mechanical trauma. This involves the removal of hair by either pulling it out by the roots or breaking it off, and both of these actions can remove a great deal more hair than you might expect. Any hair style or styling procedure that puts tension on the hair can slowly pull it out by the roots. Examples of this include wearing the hair in braids or a pony tail and wrapping it tightly around oversized hair rollers. Combing, brushing, and ratting usually don't create enough tension to pull the hair out by the roots, but they can all break off large numbers of hairs if done too vigorously.

Although contrary to the popular traditions of hair care, any combing or brushing in excess of that needed to arrange the hair is of no benefit at all, and may even relieve the head of some valuable foliage. The type of styling instrument can also make a difference; combs with sharp small teeth and stiff nylon brushes will break off more hair than blunt large-toothed combs and animal hair brushes. Even scalp massage, if overdone, can remove some hair. None of these manipulations improves the health of the hair or scalp. So why bother doing more than is absolutely necessary? The injudicious use of heat can also be bad for the hair. Curling irons, hair dryers, and the newer hot curlers and hot combs all weaken hair and make it more susceptible to mechanical trauma.

The quality or condition of the hair is important, not only for the appearance's sake, but in determining how much hair stays on the head. This is because damaged hair is much more fragile than healthy hair and can be easily broken off by scratching or one of the mechanical traumas. A cardinal rule of hair care is that poor-quality or damaged hair, like any other invalid, should always be treated as gently as possible.

Although environmental factors, such as sunlight, can affect hair quality to a slight extent, 99 per cent of all severe hair damage is caused by the application of chemicals. Waving solutions, bleaches, dyes, and hair straighteners are the worst offenders. Damaged hair not only breaks more easily than healthy hair, but it is dry, lifeless, and hard to manage. A damaged hair, if examined under a microscope, will show cracks in the shaft, split ends, and a surface that looks like a shingle roof after a hailstorm. It seems to be increasingly difficult these days to find an adult female with undamaged hair that has a completely normal texture. Although it's strictly a matter of personal opinion, I sometimes wonder whether the effects women achieve with chemicals are worth the price they have to pay in terms of texture loss.

The signs of poor-quality hair are unmistakable, and the diagnosis usually makes itself. Since the damage in all likelihood is self-inflicted and there are only a limited number of possible causes, the offending agent or agents should not be too hard to identify. The remedy is also relatively uncomplicated. Damaged hair can always be restored to its original state simply by discontinuing any abuses and letting it grow out. This may be quite a serious blow, of course, to the woman for whom waving and bleaching have become a way of life.

At this point, the reader may feel that the enumeration of all these things that can affect the hair is about as interesting as last week's grocery list. But a comprehensive checklist is unavoidable in dealing with hair problems, because tracking them down is essentially a process of elimination. The first thing to establish is whether or not a problem even exists. A change in hair quality is obvious, but a suspected hair-loss problem is much more difficult to confirm, particularly if there is no visible thinning. An extra hair or two found on the comb or brush may mean nothing more than a temporary shift in the metabolism, and new hairs may be coming in as fast as the old ones are coming out.

It should be kept in mind that the average person will lose from 40 to 100 hairs a day; some are caught by the comb or brush, but the majority fall unnoticed to the ground. The most important thing is whether the rate of loss is increasing or remaining stable. A simple test to determine this can be made by combing the hair out over a white towel at the same time every day using an equal number of strokes. The number of hairs that fall to the towel or adhere to the comb are then counted. A record of this daily loss should be kept for a period of at least six weeks. If it appears to be increasing, there is a good chance that a hair-loss problem does exist. A thorough investigation is an absolute necessity in all cases, because hair loss is often due to several interdependent factors, rather than just a single, isolated cause. For instance, the man with hereditary hair loss and a woman who rolls her hair every night will both lose more hair if they also have thyroid disease or if itchy dandruff is present. A hair-loss problem cannot be completely solved until all the contributing factors are found and eliminated, regardless of how large or small a part they play.

A general physical examination should have first priority, with particular attention being given to the glandular status and health of the scalp. If no abnormality is found, or if some scalp or internal disease is discovered for which appropriate treatment is instituted, then the physician's job is done. The rest of the investigation is up to the individual if the problem persists. If it does, then the next step is to reduce all forms of mechanical trauma to a bare minimum for a period of at least two months. Realistically speaking, it is impossible for a person to give up all styling manipulations and still appear in public, so if heat or chemicals are used on the hair, they should also be dispensed with during this period. The reason for this is that even minimal amounts of brushing and combing may perpetuate a loss problem by breaking off hairs weakened by heat or chemical damage.

If the results are all negative up to this point and if the loss continues after a period of abstention from trauma, heat, and chemicals, then the situation is in-

deed serious. This means that the problem is either
due to heredity or falls into the 'ideopathic' category.
Since nothing can be done in either case to regrow
the hair, differentiation between the two is strictly
academic. Any regrowth of hair, if it ever occurs, will
be spontaneous and not through any human efforts.
The man in this situation may face total baldness and
the woman, a very sparsely covered head. Even if the
loss is of the 'ideopathic' type and the process eventually reverses itself, the hair may never again regain its
original thickness.

The unfortunate person who finds himself in this
fix is always despairing and sometimes near-hysterical,
but there are a number of things that can be done to
partially compensate for the loss. The most obvious is
to sweep the whole problem under the rug, so to
speak, and get a wig or hairpiece. I shall only point
out that the hair-goods industry has come a long way
in the last few years, and those unfamiliar with its
progress are often pleasantly surprised by the wide
range of modern hair products and special services
now available.

If this solution is not appealing, the next approach
is to try to get more mileage out of whatever hair is
left. For one thing, dyeing the hair a darker colour
will give the illusion of thicker hair. A new and
interesting approach, with several possible applications in cases of hair loss, is the use of shampoos, conditioners, and hair dressings containing protein. This
substance has the ability to attach itself to the hair
surface, and the use of one of these products results in
each individual hair being coated with a film of pro-

tein. This increases the diameter or thickness of each hair, giving the impression that the head has more hair than it actually does. This protein film can also serve another very useful purpose where such things as waving solutions and bleaches continue to be used. These chemicals are always indirectly responsible for at least some hair loss, and protein can help protect those hairs that would ordinarily be damaged and broken off. Nearly every product on the market uses the same kind of protein (collagen protein), so brand names are unimportant. Start with one of the shampoos. If you don't get the desired results, add a protein conditioner or hair dressing. You can always tell when to stop. If you are using too much protein, the hair will become matted and hard to comb. Protein is a good example of a cosmetic ingredient that is great for one application, yet useless for another. As we have seen, it does nothing for MP films.

Finally, any nonprotein conditioning agent that makes hair more manageable, such as a cream rinse, will save some additional hair by reducing the amount of mechanical trauma needed to untangle, comb, and style.

There is a new and very successful surgical approach for the man who has a large area of bare skin on the top of his head. This procedure is actually a series of minor operations involving the relocation of scalp hair from the actively growing fringe to the hairless areas. Plugs of skin containing from four to ten hairs are surgically removed from the sides and back and transplanted to the bald scalp. Even though these hairs are moved to a completely barren area, they will continue to grow at a normal rate. The front part of the scalp is always treated first, and this new hair can be combed back to cover the intervening void as soon as it becomes long enough. The entire scalp can eventually be made to grow hair by this method, although only a very small area can be covered at each session. The process is tedious and time-consuming, but most men who have undergone hair transplantation are delighted with the results.

A full head of hair in good condition requires very little in the way of routine care. This may seem surprising at first, considering the cleansing, MP film, and thinning requirements of the skin, and the fact that the hair, after all, is just a specialized extension of the skin's outer layer. But the hair itself has physical characteristics that are quite different from those of its rather delicate parent. It is a great deal tougher than the skin and is hardly affected at all by dirt and pollutants, so a daily cleansing is not necessary. Once a week is sufficient, but twice or three times a week is permissible if chemicals are not used on the hair and the scalp tends to be oily. I always recommend Johnson's Baby Shampoo for routine hair care. It contains a special cleansing ingredient that makes it extremely mild. The hair's response to moisturization is negligible, and it requires little protection, sunlight being the only real environmental threat. Thinning the hair, of course, is synonymous with cutting it. Just because the hair requires less routine care than the skin doesn't mean it can be abused with impunity or that a hair loss problem can be ignored. Most of us don't realize how much the hair does for our appearance until it's going or gone.

The hands and nails are subject to some special problems that never trouble the face and hair, and they usually require special attention. This is because the average person exposes the hands and nails to soaps or detergents at least a dozen times a day in course of bathing, washing dishes, housekeeping, etc. This is entirely too much cleansing for these areas to tolerate indefinitely, and sooner or later they react in some manner. Red, dry, rough hands and brittle, splitting, separated nails are the results. Often, the skin signs will worsen and proceed to hand eczema, an ugly rash that requires medical treatment.

Fruit and vegetable juices invariably aggravate this situation, as do many of the household chemical products, such as furniture polishes, metal cleaners, sanitizers, etc. To make matters worse, the nails are further damaged by contact with polishes, cuticle removers, nail hardeners, and artificial nails.

The solution to these problems lies in either avoiding all the above irritants or furnishing the hands and nails some kind of physical protection. This means wearing gloves. However, you can't just throw on a pair of gloves and see all your hand and nail problems disappear. There are some definite rules regarding the wearing of gloves. If you don't know these rules and observe them, the gloves will make your problems worse instead of better.

First, remove any rings. These should never be worn inside gloves. The gloved hand has two enemies, soiled glove linings and trapped sweat. Either of these things can rapidly worsen an existing hand or nail condition, and precautions must be taken against their occurrence. Buying lined gloves is not the answer. The linings soon become dirty, and it is almost impossible to wash them. In addition, built-in linings absorb very little sweat and don't dry quickly enough. I always recommend getting rubber gloves a size too large, and then wearing light cotton gloves under them. This way, the insides of the rubber gloves stay clean, the hands stay dry, and the cotton gloves can be washed when they get dirty. Instead of rubber gloves, you can now buy thin, disposable plastic gloves by the box or roll. They allow greater dexterity, but they are more expensive.

When wearing gloves, try to stay out of hot water. I mean this literally. When the hands are covered, heat causes a tremendous outpouring of sweat, and a layer of warm sweat next to the skin can be almost as irritating as a detergent. This difficulty can be circumvented, at times, by first soaking dishes in hot water and then finishing them in cool water. Long-handled brushes and mops are helpful in situations where you must clean something immersed in hot water.

Finally, always limit your glove-wearing to no more than thirty minutes at a time. Covered hands always perspire to some extent, so remove the gloves occasionally and give the hands a chance to dry. Always rinse the hands in cool water and dry with a towel after removing the gloves.

This usually solves the skin problems, but the nails may continue to be brittle, splitting, and separated. If they do, and you have stayed away from the nail and cuticle products mentioned above, you should consult a physician. Persistent nail problems are often the first sign of some internal condition. There is also the possibility that the nails themselves may be diseased rather than damaged. In either case, medical treatment is necessary to restore them to health.

Whatever you do, don't waste your time taking gelatin. In my student days, I took part in a scientific investigation designed to evaluate the effect of gelatin on nail problems. It was my job to dispense bottles of capsules labelled 'A' and 'B.' One of these letters designated the gelatin, the other sugar, and I wasn't told which was which. (This is known as a double-blind study. Under these conditions, the clinical observer's emotions and prejudices can't affect the final results.) At the conclusion of the study, about half the people in each of my groups were convinced they saw some definite improvement in their nails. This impression pretty much anticipated the official results. It was a draw, and the 'A' and 'B' bottles were judged about equal in therapeutic value. So, if you ever find yourself seized by an irresistible urge to take something for your nails, try sugar. It's cheaper and, according to my experience, gives about the same results as gelatin.

ELEVEN

EPILOGUE

'In my youth,' said the sage,
   As he shook his grey locks,
'I kept all my limbs very supple
   By the use of this ointment—
One shilling the box—
   Allow me to sell you a couple?'

               Lewis Carroll,
               Alice's Adventures in Wonderland

The previous chapter brings us completely up to date on the art of looking younger. We have come a long way, and there is every reason to expect continued progress in the years ahead. I am convinced, however, that we will never have the very best products and methods an advanced technology can offer without some form of increased regulatory control of the cosmetic industry, including a set of uniform standards that must be met by all manufacturers. I further believe that unless some basic changes are made in the way skin-care products are sold, the consumer will never be able to utilize them to their best advantage, no matter how much the products themselves may improve.

The reforms needed to remedy this situation lie, for the most part, in the areas of product information and product evaluation. Essentially, modified versions of the same controls and standards now used for internally administered drugs should be applied to skin-care products. Although some of the more progressive cosmetic companies are already moving in this direction, the industry as a whole will never adopt these reforms without government action.

The most immediate problem concerns product information. We not only need a great deal more factual information on skin-care products, but misrepresentations and inaccuracies must be eliminated. The key to solving this problem is revised product labelling. Given only the meagre and ofttimes inaccurate information supplied with most products, it is difficult for anyone, dermatologist, cosmetologist, or consumer, to evaluate a product or match it to a particular skin. If you want to become thoroughly and completely bewildered, walk into the cosmetic department of any store and spend an hour reading the labels. The different descriptions and claims are confusing even to the professional, so the average consumer hardly stands a chance. There is a very good reason why many companies try to give you as little factual information as possible. They know that people are easily attracted to the mysterious and exotic, and that a large segment of the public can be counted on to consistently pass up the simple and practical for something with an aura of magic about it. The industry as a whole has done little to discourage this attitude, and some companies show no hesitation in exploiting it to the limit. This kind of fraud is usually justified on the grounds that what the consumer really buys is hope, and supplying this is the seller's only responsibility. It is becoming increasingly difficult to rationalize this kind of attitude in today's consumer-oriented society. Fortunately there seems to be an increasing public awareness of this whole problem. Legislation is being considered that would require the listing of all cosmetic ingredients on the label. This is a vital first step, but it doesn't go far enough. We also need to know more about the physical specifications of skin care products, and what they actually do to the skin.

The information furnished with skin care products should be concise and accurate. As things stand now, those responsible for the labelling, advertising, and selling of these products are either surprisingly ignorant of the facts, or by virtue of longstanding traditions, feel they have an unlimited licence to exercise their imaginations. Inaccurate, exaggerated, and misleading statements are collectively called 'puffery' in the trade, a term much less likely to disturb the conscience than the correct one.

The second part of this regulatory approach should be the enforcement of stricter rules covering the evaluation of new products and the use of new, unproven ingredients. New products and ingredients should not only undergo more thorough testing prior to release, but a manufacturer should be required to verify any claims and furnish proof of effectiveness. In this way, the consumer would be assured that there were no undue hazards connected with a product's use, and that it would perform as advertised. Under the present system, products are being marketed with certain highly controversial ingredients that are probably of no benefit whatsoever.

What would be the practical results of all these reforms? The most immediate change would be a marked improvement in both the selection and utilization of skin care products by the consumer. Eventually, the overall quality of the products themselves would be greatly improved. Since they would be sold on the basis of merit and proven effectiveness, rather than creative advertising, those companies that depended on 'puffery' to sell substandard merchandise would have to change their ways or go out of business. Old products would have to be re-examined, and all new products and ingredients would undergo more thorough evaluation and testing prior to release. The net results would be better and safer products for the consumer.

Finally, companies would almost certainly have to give their sales personnel better training in order to compete under these conditions, and this would be of inestimable value to the consumer. Selling skin care products and advice on skin care is a highly technical business, compared to, say, selling lingerie, and the average level of sales indoctrination is pitifully low. Lacking a complete understanding of what they sell, sales persons are often forced to improvise, and the results can be wildly imaginative. Better trained, more knowledgeable personnel would mean better all-around service to the consumer, who, armed with better information, could not only buy and use skin-care products more intelligently, but play a larger part in their selection. The theory that the average person is incapable of understanding the fundamentals of good skin care is plainly untrue. However, the companies that make and sell these products obviously have a vested interest in maintaining their

advantage and keeping the consumer totally dependent on them. Although few of us really like the idea
of increased government controls, the results in this
instance would more than justify the means.

INDEX

THE JOY OF SLIMMING

MARGARET ALLAN

Here at last is a book which offers a positive approach to slimming. It tells you what you CAN eat, instead of what you CAN'T, and offers a wealth of mouth-watering recipes to prove the point.

Margaret Allan is a scientist who has made a special study of excess weight and other slimming problems. In this very special book she shuns fads and gimmicks and applies a common sense approach to the difficulties of losing weight. Superb recipes, menu suggestions, calorie and carbohydrate charts, food value tables, detailed slimming exercises and a question-and-answer section combine to make this a complete and thoroughly practical guide for all slimmers.

CORONET BOOKS

NUTRITION AND YOUR MIND

DR. GEORGE WATSON

Are you a fast oxidiser who burns his food up quickly? Or a slow one who burns it up slowly? Do you ever feel depressed, irritable or downright ill? If so, you may be suffering from the kind of brain starvation which is caused by the wrong diet. In this extraordinary new book Dr. George Watson draws on his many years of research to explain how your physical and mental health can be sensationally affected by the food you eat.

NUTRITION AND YOUR MIND explores a startling new theory about the relationship between nutrition and your health. The book also contains a questionnaire which will help you discover your own psychochemical type and a number of fascinating case histories.

CORONET BOOKS

ALSO AVAILABLE IN CORONET BOOKS

All these books are available at your local bookshop or newsagent, or can be ordered direct from the publisher. Just tick the titles you want and fill in the form below.

Prices and availability subject to change without notice.

CORONET BOOKS, P.O. Box 11, Falmouth, Cornwall.

Please send cheque or postal order, and allow the following for postage and packing:

U.K. – One book 19p plus 9p per copy for each additional book ordered, up to a maximum of 73p.

B.F.P.O. and EIRE – 19p for the first book plus 9p per copy for the next 6 books, thereafter 3p per book.

OTHER OVERSEAS CUSTOMERS – 20p for the first book and 10p per copy for each additional book.

Name ....

Address..

....